Remarkable Caregiving

Endorsements

Nancy Poland has written a compelling book that is as practical and helpful as it is inspiring and uplifting. Herein are the stories of six truly remarkable caregivers who found themselves living lives they never envisioned. There are big challenges and small victories for each caregiver, and through it all, we are reminded of the transforming nature of self-sacrificial love. Highly recommended!

Terry Weston Marsh, M.D., Mooreland, Indiana

As an estate planning attorney for 30 years, I have seen a lot. But these stories offered by Nancy Poland in *"Remarkable Caregiving"* are in every sense *"*remarkable*"*. If only I could get this book in front of all my prospective clients. I love how the author skillfully weaves in the proper and improper use estate planning tools and legal proceedings. She also powerfully portrays the secret burdens others carry while illuminating the perseverance and love of the human spirit. You will recognize a family member or even yourself in these remarkable stories.

Joe Field, Esq., Anoka, MN, Author, *Finding Joe Adams*

Caregivers are often charged with decisions where there is no right or wrong answer. *Remarkable Caregiving* provides insight into the journey and decisions of six caregivers. Each story lifted my spirits and was filled with practical information and lessons. Love was the common thread throughout the book.

Carol B. Amos, Author of *H.O.P.E. for the Alzheimer's Journey: Help, Organization, Preparation, and Education for the Road Ahead*

In nearly one-third of American households, there is an elderly person, a disabled person or someone who is ill being cared for by some other family member. And as our population ages, that startling number is sure to grow. Behind these statistics are people (moms, dads, sons, daughters, just friends) who live every day with the two basic realities of caregiving: they truly "care" for and about the person whom they have taken responsibility for, and they are constantly "giving" to the person. That includes their time, their energy, their finances, their heart and their hope. In her new book, *Remarkable Caregiving*, Nancy Poland puts faces to those statistics, sharing in-depth and up-close profiles of six stories of people in need and the people who have made the lifelong sacrifice to meet those needs. The stories cover the gamut of caregiver types, from children caring for aging and ill parents, to parents navigating life with a special needs child, to a friend helping his childhood pal navigate a debilitating illness, but the underlying love, grace and tenacity are universal. Wherever you stand in the caregiving equation--as a giver, a recipient or just a concerned family member or friend--this book will educate you, break your heart and lift your spirits with these amazing examples of how God blesses and strengthens His children during their darkest days and loneliest nights.

Ken Adkins, author of *The Silent Son: Lessons Learned from Raising a Special Needs Child*

Nancy R. Poland's latest book *Remarkable Caregiving* is a remarkable *treasure* of heart wrenching yet heartwarming stories representing the now one in five American adults providing care for a disabled or ill adult or child. A must read for anyone touched in any way by the caregiving journey, and a great way to honor and more deeply appreciate these often-unsung heroes among us.

Sue Flesch, B.S., Clinical Research Associate, Childhood Cancer Survivorship, St. Paul, MN

Nancy Poland has opened our eyes as she unfolds the heartwarming care and struggles of six caregivers who gave love, understanding and support on behalf of their loved ones as they journeyed through home care concerns. Nancy shares these diverse stories not only to validate the efforts of those who help vulnerable adults and children as they advocate to keep their dignity and independence, but to help those who are going through similar situations by offering home care check lists and questions to stimulate those hard discussions with family and friends. You will find strength as well as tears, to helpful information, as each story motivates you to read the next one where faith, individual worldviews and love for others touches our hearts.

Tery Blahut, SILS (Semi-Independent Living Service) for vulnerable handicapped adults and assistant at Life Enrichment Programs (retired)

In *"Remarkable Caregiving"* Nancy Poland has assembled an inspiring collection of caregiving stories in which the love of family and friends is evident as is the creativity and unique approach to meet each need. Families will find encouragement, ideas, and helpful resources as they walk their own caregiving journeys.

Martina Hartmark, M.D.,
Internal Medicine Physician, Minneapolis, MN

Whether life chooses you as caregiver to parent, spouse or child, or you step up to help a friend, this book shares comfort, encouragement, and lessons learned from real life hero/survivors. As a cancer survivor and later power of attorney for my mother during her dementia, I have been on both sides of caregiving. I wish I had this book then; I will share this book with my caregiver friends in the future.

Marla K. Hartson, Author, *Praise PhD: Praising God in the Middle of the Valley of Cancer*, Trainer: *Friends with Cancer: How to Help*

Step by step the stories are told, of the weak, of the brave… and of the bold. Nancy offers true life to her stories. She uses valuable tools to encourage and equip others. Sharing valuable, necessary information is a key component for the hard conversations that are inevitable. An excellent source for caregivers.

Lynn Porath, Certified Registered Nurse, St. Paul, MN

Nancy Poland truly touches the heart of the critical challenges faced by family caregivers. In six distinctive true-life scenarios spanning from infants to the elderly, she brings the reader into an empathetic understanding of dealing with the roles of stress and hope facing an effective caregiver. She also provides excellent resources to support families in meeting the demands of caring for loved ones with special needs. This is an excellent heart-warming read that brings significant awareness and insight into the dynamics of family life requiring special care for individual members. It was a true privilege reading *Remarkable Caregiving*; I am grateful it expanded my awareness of caregiving.

Merrill Kindall, Retired Pastor, Minneapolis, MN

remarkable
CAREGIVING
The Care of Family & Friends

NANCY R. POLAND

NEW YORK

LONDON • NASHVILLE • MELBOURNE • VANCOUVER

Remarkable Caregiving

The Care of Family and Friends

Published in New York, New York, by Morgan James Publishing. Morgan James is a trademark of Morgan James, LLC. www.MorganJamesPublishing.com

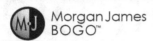

Morgan James BOGO™

A **FREE** ebook edition is available for you or a friend with the purchase of this print book.

CLEARLY SIGN YOUR NAME ABOVE

Instructions to claim your free ebook edition:
1. Visit MorganJamesBOGO.com
2. Sign your name CLEARLY in the space above
3. Complete the form and submit a photo of this entire page
4. You or your friend can download the ebook to your preferred device

ISBN 9781631955433 paperback
ISBN 9781631955440 ebook
Library of Congress Control Number: 2021933091

Cover Design by:
Megan Dillon
megan@creativeninjadesigns.com

Interior Design by:
Christopher Kirk
www.GFSstudio.com

All Scripture quotations, unless otherwise indicated, are taken from the Holy Bible, New International Version® NIV®. Copyright © 1973, 1978, 1984, 2011 by Biblica, Inc.® Used by permission. All rights reserved worldwide.

Illustrated by Nancy Muellner, nancymuellner.com

Disclaimer
While these stories relay events that actually occurred, names and identifying details have been changed to protect the privacy of individuals and businesses, with one exception. "Lutheran Social Service" is the true name of the organization in Chapter 6, used by permission.
This book is not intended as a substitute for medical, financial, or legal advice of experts. The reader should consult professionals in matters relating to these issues.

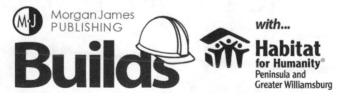

Morgan James is a proud partner of Habitat for Humanity Peninsula and Greater Williamsburg. Partners in building since 2006.

Get involved today! Visit
MorganJamesPublishing.com/giving-back

Also by Nancy R. Poland
Dancing With Lewy:
A Father Daughter Dance Before and After
Lewy Body Dementia Came to Live With Us

For the six caregivers who shared their story for this book;
you know who you are, and to you we are grateful.
Your life experiences, pain and hope
will pave the way for caregivers everywhere.

Table of Contents

Foreword

There are more than fifty-three million caregivers in America today.[1] Despite the prevalence of caregiving, family members who assume the caregiver role often feel alone, confused, and overwhelmed.

Faced with the challenge of caring for a loved one with serious and often life-threatening medical conditions, family caregivers frequently find themselves unprepared to address the complex physical, emotional, mental, financial, temporal, and spiritual implications of care.

Nevertheless, they do not give up. How do family caregivers summon the strength they need to continue supporting their loved one?

They love and they learn.

Love is what motivates family caregivers to assume new care-related responsibilities. Love leads family caregivers to sacrifice for their loved ones. Love has the ability to envelop caregivers and care receivers as they traverse through the unanticipated changes that caregiving forces upon their relationships and their lives.

Although love may be motivational, it is not enough for family caregivers to successfully meet the needs of their loved ones. Every family caregiver must also learn how to deliver care while factoring all the peculiarities of their loved one's situation. Learning thus becomes an intrinsic part of fulfilling the caregiver role. The learning process is marked by continual adaptation: as the loved one's physical, mental, emotional, environmental, financial needs change, the family caregiver must discover how to modify services and supports in the most satisfactory way.

In *Remarkable Caregiving*, Nancy R. Poland has assembled a beautiful collection of stories about caregivers who love and learn. The families presented in the following pages did not plan to become caregivers, but in each case, the emerging needs of a loved one required a change of plans. As these caregivers faced seemingly insurmountable challenges and self-doubt, it was love that fueled their desire to continue. Through their perseverance, the caregivers learned how to serve their loved ones better, revealing a measure of resourcefulness they never knew they had and a growing confidence that they were acting in the best interest of their loved ones.

Amid the sadness and adversity of their lives, these caregivers found unanticipated and at times miraculous growth. Like so many caregivers, they progressed through a range of emotions, moving from confusion, anger, or disbelief to a sense of understanding and acceptance. They often speak of the centrality of faith in their odyssey of caregiving. Their new perspectives have allowed them to share practical and inspirational advice for others, which the author (a caregiver herself) has graciously recorded for the reader.

The caregivers in this book probably would not consider themselves to be remarkable. Most likely, they would say they were just doing what had to be done to help a loved one in need, and that is certainly true. At the same time, one cannot read these stories without appreciating the strain and the selflessness of their caregiving experiences. Individually and collectively, these six stories reflect what is happening in the lives of countless other caregivers whose stories have not been published.

As a result, Nancy R. Poland has produced a book for all caregivers—past, present, and future—who are, by definition, remarkable.

Aaron Blight, Ed.D.,
Author of *When Caregiving Calls: Guidance as You Care for a Parent, Spouse, or Aging Relative*

Preface

Fiddler on the Roof
Elf on the Shelf
Santa Clause

What could I have in common with these three mythical figures?

"Fiddler on the Roof" the musical released in 1971 is based on the book by Joseph Stein. The Fiddler, perched on a roof, bears witness to Tevye in 1905 Russia as he struggles with a changing world. Along with The Fiddler, we witness Tevye's five daughters progressively move away from their family and faith as they mature and marry. Finally, they are displaced by the discriminatory pogroms in Russia.

"Elf on the Shelf" is the main character in the children's book written by Carol B. Aebersold and Chandra A. Bell, illustrated by Coe Steinwart. Families can obtain their own Elf, who moves about the house, keeping a watchful eye on the children. The Elf then reports their behavior back to Santa.

And, of course, Santa Clause sees and knows all: who is sleeping, who is awake, and who has been good and bad!

Like our mythical figures, I was able to take a peek into the lives of six individuals who agreed to be interviewed. I was hoping to satisfy my curiosity about human resilience and resourcefulness in caregiving. What makes people put their lives on hold for a family member? What drives a mother to pour unexplainable love on a child with disabilities? What is the cement holding a friendship together, expressed through years of mutual support?

I was hoping for a formula, common traits, or consistent personality types that turned these every-day people into remarkable human beings.

While six interviews do not result in a scientific conclusion, these stories led me to something I did not expect. The interviews brought laughter and tears. Their stories were gripping and emotional. Sometimes, we had to pause to catch our breaths.

What I found were whole families with ranges of emotions. People who struggled and problem-solved, finding themselves in situations they would not have chosen but to which they adapted. Freely sharing their stories and humbly providing advice for others, some fought back tears. Faith, personal worldviews, and family connections are interwoven into the fabric of these stories. All were motivated by love.

As you read these stories, may you also be moved by these brave individuals. To my six friends, old and new, along with the others who contributed to the narrative, thank you for sharing your stories and your hearts.

Chapter 1
The Kidnapping Plot

"Things turn out best for those who make the best of the way things turn out."
– Jack Buck

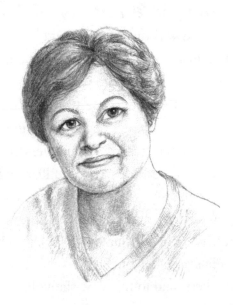

Introduction

When I asked my friend Cynthia if she would be willing to share her caregiving story, she enthusiastically agreed. A smart, analytical businesswoman, one would never think she would find herself in the midst of a legal quagmire. Cynthia loves her family and takes after her hardworking dad. Now, she will forever wonder how they found themselves in such a situation.

Cynthia also adored her savvy, hardworking mom, and maybe she did not recognize the signs of her mom's decline because her mom had been so competent and was always there for her children and husband. Cynthia still speaks with regret and shares her story in hopes of helping other families avoid some of the pitfalls this family encountered.

Life Learning in a Family of Eleven

Cynthia is hardworking, sincere, and born to be a caretaker. The eldest child in a large family, Cynthia is nurturing and caring yet organized with a take-charge personality.

When I first met Cynthia, she was on a committee hosting a convention where I was a speaker. I forgot my handouts in my room on the other side of the convention center. Without a thought, Cynthia asked for my room key and marched off to gather my materials. She would walk to the end of the earth for a friend; if you could meet her, you would love her.

As a Certified Public Accountant (CPA), Cynthia served several cities as the Finance Director. She has always used her financial skills to help others, and to this day, she volunteers to keep books for nonprofits. She is savvy in the business and financial world.

So, what would possess Cynthia, an honest, law-abiding citizen, to illegally kidnap a woman and cross three state lines?

Cynthia's work ethic and family loyalty came from her parents, Rob and Margaret. They married in 1955 after Rob served in the Marines during the Korean War. Living first in a suburb of Minneapolis, they later bought ninety acres in a small Minnesota town as their family of six outgrew the urban house. Their family later grew by three more for a total of nine children.

Rob and Margaret had what was called at that time a "mixed faith marriage." Rob in his early days was a non-practicing Protestant, and Margaret was a strong Catholic. Her mother faithfully took the children to church every Sunday, volunteered at church events, and belonged to the women's group. In his later years, Cynthia's father became active in the Baptist faith but never attended church regularly. Nevertheless, he had a strong faith and always had his Bible nearby.

Cynthia describes her dad as "smart, kind and caring, although he did not always demonstrate his feelings. I knew he loved me, and he adored my mom. Resourceful and able to figure out how to build almost anything, Dad made a living developing and fixing packaging machinery. Dad had an engineering mind and was self-taught. He built my first computer from scratch when computers were just coming into their own."

Cynthia says her mom kept busy with their large family. She describes her mom as "kind, thoughtful, loving. She excelled at being a homemaker. Mom was a skilled seamstress, cook, and baker. She was also resourceful. With nine kids, we did not have a lot of money, but we never went hungry."

Cynthia thought for a minute before continuing, "We did have unusual foods at times, like eggplant parmesan, which only one brother liked—we think it was because of the crunchy coating. Once she made corn chowder, which none of us liked. Then there was the time she fed us liver, but only once as no one ate that either. I think someone must have given us the meat. Ick! We had a lot of 'hotdishes.' You know a hotdish can feed a lot of people, like the one made with noodles, ground beef, and spaghetti sauce.

"We were not picky eaters. If you went hungry, she let us know she was not making two meals! At one point, we were on food stamps for a short time, and Mom made sure to go to a grocery store where no one knew her because she was embarrassed."

Retirement

In 2003, the hardworking Rob approached his much-deserved retirement. At the same time, he was contacted by a developer who wanted to buy their entire property. Instead, Rob and one of his sons made plans to develop the property themselves. There were a number of delays and problems due to the political nature of township boards, but finally, the ninety acres were developed into twelve beautiful lots ready to be put on the market. Unfortunately, the market made a major downturn then.

The lots sold, albeit slowly, but the sale of the lots provided Rob and his wife the needed income to purchase a new home for their retirement.

One sunny spring, Rob and Margaret went on a vacation with Cynthia and her husband, Tony, to a timeshare near Branson, Missouri. The people in the communities loved the area and spoke highly of it, promoting the neighborhood as a great place to retire. The area had a high number of retirees living there with great medical facilities.

"No," said Rob. "This is nice, but it is just is not for us. Let's keep looking."

Margaret smiled and nodded in agreement.

Rob and Margaret drove up and down through the hills of Missouri hunting for the right property. They fell in love with a small town forty-five minutes from Branson. After a fact-finding trip, they bought property in the rural, rolling hills.

Excited, they began to organize a lifetime of possessions. Rob did most of the work while Margaret picked through and resorted items. Rob did not like to ask his children for help, having once told Cynthia, "It is easier to do it myself instead of arguing with your brothers."

With equipment capable of moving a thousand pounds, Rob, independent and determined, packed up all of their worldly goods. Boxes were carefully placed into the moving truck, and machinery was placed on trailers. Rob took every piece of equipment he owned. The couple headed to Missouri, 850 miles from home, for their next phase of life. After their busy lives, Rob and Margaret enjoyed the peace and quiet of the country.

The next town over had about 2,500 people. There they could grocery shop, bank, and get gas. Medical care was in Branson, a lengthy drive through the winding roads of the Ozarks. Even with the milder climate, they still had to contend with some snow, and often, the hills iced over in the winter.

It seemed like a good idea—until life dealt them a different hand. More on that later.

Cynthia's dad later admitted purchasing the property in the rural area became a serious challenge for them by conceding, "It may have been better if we had moved to a bigger town."

In addition, it was at least an eleven-hour drive from most of their kids, other than one daughter who was in the next state over but still a four-hour drive away. This daughter eventually moved back to Minnesota, so that lifeline was lost.

During and after the move, Cynthia noticed her mom was having memory issues.

Her mom would ask, "Honey, do you have my camera?"

"No, Mom, you took it with you," Cynthia replied.

"I'm sure you have it!"

"Mom, did you look in your desk where you used to keep it? Or your dresser drawer?"

"Of course," said Mom, "I am sure you have it."

Rob confirmed they did have the camera.

A few days later, her mom would call again about the "lost" camera.

Another time, Margaret called Cynthia, saying her youngest brother was taking her Royal Dalton collectible figurines or sewing machines. She told Cynthia that she was sure he was giving them to his girlfriend so he could "make points." Cynthia would go back and forth with her mother correcting and arguing with her, asking why she would think her son would take her things.

Cynthia now wishes she had known more about dementia. Instead of arguing or correcting her mom, she would have gone along with her or redirected her questions. However, like many of us, we go about our daily lives and are easily caught off guard when a little-understood predicament descends on our family. At that time, Cynthia attributed her mom's forgetfulness to the move, thinking her mother was a little disoriented.

Her mom's forgetfulness got worse, but she was mild-mannered and usually pleasant. Rob vowed to take care of his beloved wife.

Because Cynthia's parents were so far away, they would only see each other a couple of times a year. Rob and Margaret remained fiercely independent and rarely asked for help from their children. With their kids so far away, no one realized how serious the situation was becoming.

The Biggest Regret

Not only did Rob and Margaret's kids have to deal with their parent's health issues from afar, but Cynthia was also soon to find out how more of her dad's decisions would affect her ability to take care of her parents.

Having never dealt with seniors and their legal needs, and knowing her dad was a savvy businessman, it did not occur to Cynthia, or any of her siblings, to get involved with her parents' legal documents. With regret, Cynthia told me, "Knowing what I know today, I would have been more proactive in making sure my dad had their legal affairs in order."

Both of her parents had wills, and her dad had a durable power of attorney document for financial purposes. He also had a healthcare directive; her mom did not.

> A healthcare directive is a written document spelling out your wishes about your healthcare. You can name a person ("agent") to decide on your care or access your medical records if you are unable to do so. You can also name an alternative agent.

(See Appendix 1, "Financial and Legal Review" for a list of financial and legal considerations and more general descriptions.)

To this day, Cynthia does not understand why her father obtained a healthcare directive for himself but not for his wife. She thinks her dad signed his wife's name to get around not having the healthcare directive in place, which would have been needed to obtain or transfer her medical records.

Ten years after the move, Cynthia's dad's health started to decline. In the late 1990s, he had a quintuple heart bypass. In 2013, he was diagnosed with leukemia brought on by age, and he had to drive to Branson for treatments. He also had heart disease, type II diabetes, and developed stage IV kidney disease and cellulitis in one leg, along with having a mild stroke at one point. Cynthia and her husband, Tony, went down to see her parents more often, as did some of her siblings, but it took time to figure out how seriously her parents' health affected their daily lives.

One time her dad let it slip he had rolled the Jeep on the icy roads. Margaret was temporarily in a nursing home for two weeks. After she came home Rob vowed, "I will never again put your mom in a nursing home as it would be as if she was gone."

After hearing this story, on the drive home, Cynthia lamented to her husband about the state of her parents' declining health. She drove with a wrinkled brow, developing a headache on the long Interstate 35 drive through the flat plains of Missouri, Iowa, and Minnesota.

Cynthia and her siblings would say, "Dad, I think you should move back to Minnesota where we can help you."

Strong-willed and independent, Rob would say, "No, we like it here. We are fine. I can take care of your mom, and we have everything we need."

Reluctantly, the topic was dropped.

Legal Limbo

Cynthia traveled down to Missouri more often to care for her parents. Sometimes, Tony went along, but because he is blind, she did all of the driving. At times, another family member would accompany her if Tony could not.

Cynthia was scheduled for carpal tunnel surgery. Since she had to take time off work to recover, she decided it would be a good time to drive to see her parents. Unfortunately, she used her hand too much while driving, and it was reinjured. Cynthia had to have the procedure redone, and the surgery was much more difficult and painful the second time. She wished that she had rescheduled the original hand surgery for after her trip to visit her parents.

As her dad's health declined, it became more difficult for him to care for his wife and himself. In 2014, while mowing the lawn, Rob suffered another stroke. He was alert enough to call 911 for help. The ambulance took both parents to the hospital, and Cynthia was called. She jumped in her car with her sister Julie, making the ten-hour trip down in record time, planning to get their parents healthy again and settled back into their home.

Julie, not understanding the legalities involved, wanted to know if she could have an advance on her inheritance. She said it was because she and her husband had limited financial resources and needed money. Cynthia just shook her head, disappointed that Julie would be thinking about her inheritance right after their dad had a stroke.

Cynthia and Julie arrived at the hospital, exhausted from the trip, and not knowing what to expect. They were told neither parent could go home. Their mother could not go home because of her advanced dementia, and their dad's health had declined too much, exacerbated by taking care of his wife for over ten years as her health continued to decline. Their parents needed to go into a nursing home.

Cynthia discovered that an adult who is unable to make their own decisions cannot go into a nursing facility without a healthcare directive or court intervention. It was too late for Margaret to sign such a directive because she was not considered mentally competent.

Cynthia, even while exasperated, understood the reasoning. "This goes way back to the 'olden days.' When a person wanted to get rid of a spouse, they would declare them insane and 'pack them away' to languish in an institution. Over time, the laws changed, and a person cannot be placed in a facility without oversight."

Cynthia was told they would have to get a court order for guardianship of her mom. The social worker gave Cynthia several names of local attorneys who could assist with getting the legal papers in order. The hospital found a nursing home that agreed to take Margaret, contingent on obtaining a guardianship order from the court. Margaret was settled in the nursing home's dementia unit while they waited for the court order.

The following day, Cynthia's father was placed in the same nursing home. With his healthcare directive in place, the process went smoothly.

Cynthia did not know anyone in the small community, so she just picked one of the attorney names provided by the hospital. It turned out he was not the best choice she could have made.

With a slight roll of her eyes and shake of her head, Cynthia reported, "A lot of snafus happened."

The attorney filed the petition, and a court date was set for two weeks later.

Communication with the attorney was sparse. Cynthia briefly met with the paralegal because the attorney was not available. While there, she asked the paralegal if she could use the restroom. The paralegal pointed the way. Cynthia said, "To get to the bathroom, I had to go through the attorney's office. That should have been my first clue that this office lacked professionalism!"

Cynthia was busy running to the nursing home to check on her parents, communicating with her siblings, and trying to figure out their bills. She then returned to Minnesota to wait for the court date.

The paralegal emailed Cynthia, which she quickly read, missing the statement at the bottom about meeting the attorney at his office prior to the court hearing.

The meeting was in the county seat in a nearby town. Upon arriving back in Missouri, Cynthia, accompanied by her sister Julie, parked the car by a large building and saw an older man in a rocking chair on the other side of Main Street.

Cynthia got out of the car, walked partway across the street, and asked, "Sir, is that the courthouse?"

"Yes, it is."

Cynthia tucked her portfolio containing her paperwork under her arm and strode across the street. Julie trailed a couple of steps behind. Cynthia's neatly coifed dark hair stayed in place, although she could already feel the sweat accumulating on her back. She realized she should have dressed cooler for the Missouri summer.

Having never been to court before, Cynthia was unaware of the process. She looked around and sat on a bench in the hall, waiting for the attorney to arrive. Where was he?

Then in walked the man she had questioned across the street. He asked if she was Cynthia and then introduced himself as the attorney. She thought, *Didn't you realize I was the only stranger in town this morning, and I had to have been your client?* But she did not want to antagonize him by stating her thoughts.

"Now, um…let's see," the attorney started. "This is about your mother…" He started going over items that could come up in court, but before he was finished, it was their turn to go into the courtroom.

As a result of not meeting with the attorney ahead of time, Cynthia was unprepared for the court appearance.

On the witness stand, her attorney asked her, "What would you like to do?"

Without thinking, Cynthia replied, "What do you think I should do?"

The judge scolded her, telling her she should not be asking the questions, and she should have been better prepared. Cynthia was taken back by being "chewed out."

The flustered attorney tried to salvage the situation. He said, "Your Honor, Cynthia is a CPA."

The judge retorted, "I do not care if she's a CPA. I am looking out for a vulnerable adult."

After a short questioning session, the hearing was over. The determination would come at a later date. Cynthia was sure she would not be approved for guardianship of her mom.

Cynthia accompanied the attorney back to his office.

He said, "In your mother's condition, it would be best if she died."

Cynthia was shocked and vowed to immediately find another attorney once the guardianship process was finalized.

The attorney, wiping his brow with his damp handkerchief, said he would let her know when the judgment was rendered.

Cynthia later said this was the most unprofessional office and attorney she had ever come across. "This was not just a small-town attorney's office. I lived in a small town for many years. It was their incompetence and uncaring attitude."

The only positive outcome was that Julie, having observed the court process, did not ask again about her share of the inheritance. She understood the seriousness of the situation.

Twenty-One Days

Cynthia knew her parents' physical needs would be taken care of in the nursing home, so she headed back home. She was relieved to arrive back in Minnesota where she sought refuge with her loving husband. Tony knew how to help her sort out her fears and her feelings. Smart and resourceful, he was set up with a complete computer system for the blind. Tony researched alternatives and solutions for Cynthia's family situation.

Cynthia needed to catch up with work, sort through the pile of mail at home, and figure out the next steps for her parents' situation. But sooner than she had hoped, it became apparent she would need to go back to tend to her parents, so back down I-35 Cynthia headed.

After the guardianship fiasco, Cynthia knew they would need a different attorney, so she asked others for a referral. This time, she found a good elder-care attorney who was more professional and knowledgeable and a better communicator, in addition to being familiar with how the laws in Missouri applied to Cynthia's parents.

Cynthia was awarded "guardianship" for her mom. She was happy to have this win, but her optimism quickly faded when she discovered this did not mean she had the authority to decide on her mom's care.

"You do not answer to the family; you answer to the courts," Cynthia lamented.

Cynthia had to record every cent of money spent on her mom, and she filed monthly financial reports with the court. Permission would be needed for major decisions concerning her mom.

Cynthia's dad had gone into the nursing home on June 26th where he received nursing care and physical therapy. A couple of times, Christine brought Rob home to visit and help sort through their items. But once Rob stayed home too long and missed his physical therapy appointment.

The nursing staff said, "If your dad misses any more appointments, Medicare may not pay for his care. He has to show commitment and improvement."

After that, the family was more diligent about getting him back on time after home visits.

Cynthia's mom was still in the dementia unit, and although she could not care for herself, Medicare would not cover her costs. Cynthia paid for her mom's care out of her parents' money.

With nine siblings you would expect disagreements. However Cynthia said there was only one intense friction, which was when her parents were first placed in the nursing home. Her sister Mary had called to check in and began questioning decisions on their care. Cynthia, totally exhausted, "lost it" and yelled at her sister. Cynthia tried to hang up on her, but her cell phone did not disconnect. Later they both apologized, understanding the stress everyone was under, and having learned the power of forgiveness from their parents.

The stress of running around with all of the appointments and planning would wear out anyone, and Cynthia was no exception. As she looked around her parents' home, tears sprung to her eyes. Usually, the strong one in the family, she felt spent, as if she had nothing left inside.

Fortunately, her brother Steven and his partner Mateo came just when she was at the breaking point. This boosted her spirits, and together, the three of them began to clean out their parents' household belongings—under their dad's watchful eye. At first, useless items were thrown in the garbage can, but it was only thirty gallons, and they were not allowed to overfill it. So they obtained a dumpster, but only made a small dent in cleaning out the house.

Rob realized he would not be coming home anytime soon, so Cynthia began talking about getting him and her mother back to Minnesota and closer to seven of their children. Rob agreed and worked more diligently with his kids to sort through their belongings.

After a couple of weeks, Rob continued to get weaker, and the nursing home staff warned that he might not live much longer. Several family members came down to see their parents. Cynthia's youngest sister Susan was a hard worker and stayed to help Cynthia sort through their parents' belongings. Steven and his Mateo came back to visit and to help, as did Cynthia's brother Mark.

They were cleaning out a lifetime of their parents' possessions—dishes, tools, letters, and books. When Rob and Margaret moved, they had packed and moved multiple boxes and crates. Between Margaret's dementia and Rob's physical decline, they never got around to unpacking most of the containers.

Cynthia and her siblings did not know what to do with all of their parents' stuff. The closest secondhand store was 30 miles away, and the largest vehicle they had was Rob's Jeep.

Cynthia hauled a lot of old computer and printer parts home to recycle at her county recycling center. She said, "They did not believe all this stuff was personal. They thought I was unloading equipment from a business, which was not allowed in the local recycling center."

Multiple storage sheds stood on the property, including one that was full of fabric. Margaret, an accomplished seamstress, had worked part-time for a fabric store in her later years. The family often joked, "Mom took her pay in fabric."

In mid-July, time moved like a slow-motion picture. Cynthia was once more back in Minnesota to her job and home. Her brother Mark was still in Missouri with their parents. Cynthia had barely been home, and on July 16th—only twenty days after her dad entered the nursing home—Mark called to say their dad had taken a turn for the worse. Cynthia immediately headed back to Missouri with her sister Susan to provide support to Mark and see their parents. On July 17th, Rob revived, so they brought him pizza from his favorite restaurant for lunch.

Thinking Rob was improving, they decided to get rid of the fabric the next day. Boxes of fabric were set on the curb with a sign, "Free fabric."

Cynthia says, "It was like cats on seafood. People came from all over the township to get the free fabric. One lady filled up her car so much she didn't have room for her kid."

Friends called friends, and the cars lined up. It was the best way to get rid of a shed full of fabric. The people in the area did not have a lot of money and were grateful for the material. Margaret would have been pleased with how her children disposed of the fabric.

Late that afternoon, the phone rang. Rob was doing worse. Cynthia and her brother headed to the nursing home once again, leaving Susan to finish the fabric giveaway. Soon, they realized their dad was not going to rally.

Hospice was called, and a hospice volunteer sat with the family during Rob's last hours. On July 18th, Rob left the cares of this earth.

Rob was brought back to Minnesota to be cremated. Cynthia points out cremation in Missouri would have been only $895, including a plastic box for his ashes. However, when they arranged for him to be cremated in Minnesota, they found the cost was $1,695, plus an additional $12 for the box. Cynthia thought, *location is everything, even when it comes to cremation!*

A Sad Goodbye

The nursing home strongly suggested they tell Margaret about her husband's death.

Cynthia said, "I didn't know why. What was the point?"

But she conceded and gently told her mom her beloved Rob had died. No reaction came from Margaret. She just continued to stare straight ahead with blank eyes. However, the nursing home staff later told Cynthia that her mom was agitated for several days afterward. She knew in her heart that her soulmate was gone.

As they prepared to leave, Cynthia stopped to say a painful goodbye to her mom.

Cynthia said, "I love you, Mom."

Clear as a bell, her mom said, "I love you too."

For a brief moment, her mom was back. Cynthia left the nursing home crying. She said, "Leaving Mom alone in a different state in the care of others was one of the hardest things I ever had to do."

After a brief trip at home, Cynthia, her brother Mark, and sister Susan headed back to spend time with their mom. They also continued dealing with the household goods, knowing their mom would not be coming back. It was a sizzling hot summer for people used to the northern climate.

This time, her brother brought a trailer. The household items were sorted, and her brother packed up the trailer to bring home items other family members wanted. He had clearly inherited his dad's ability to sort and organize. Cynthia could not believe all he was able to pack into the trailer.

There were many other items to be dealt with. Her dad's cancer medication came in the mail. The cost (before insurance) was over $6,000 a month, and the central pharmacy would not just stop sending the medication on Cynthia's request. She needed to take the medication back to the clinic; they were able to put a stop to the order.

When they cleaned out their parent's medicine cabinet, they came up with a full bag of medications, vitamins, and ointments. Cynthia took the bag to the medicine drop-off at the local police station. As she was leaving, she saw the sign that said, "No ointments." "Oops," was her reaction as she pulled away.

Cynthia gathered half a grocery bag full of diabetes supplies. After finding no one in Missouri who would take the items, she brought them back to Minnesota and gave the bag to a sister who knew people who could use the supplies.

They filled several dumpsters with stuff not worth saving. Other items were sold in a moderately successful garage sale, and they gave away what they could not sell, fulfilling the needs of many people in the area. Cynthia knew her parents would be happy knowing others benefited from what they had accumulated. Once the items were out of the house, Cynthia arranged for the house and carpet to be cleaned in preparation for the sale.

Cynthia also took care of their financial matters but quickly ran into resistance. Even though Cynthia had been the personal representative via her dad's power of attorney document, that power went away when he died. She had to wait for the death certificate to be issued by the state.

Between the death certificate and the will, she was able to start dealing with the business matters. For one, Rob had squirreled away money in a number of different banks. Cynthia said, "He had money all over. Finally, having all of the correct documents, it took three trips to get the money out of just one of the banks."

During the summer of 2014 while all of this was taking place, Cynthia made numerous trips back and forth between Minnesota and Missouri. She used a lot of vacation time from work taking care of her parents, handling legal details, getting the house and storage building cleaned out, and working to dispose of fifty-nine years' worth of belongings. She figures she used over three-hundred hours of her vacation time that summer.

Cynthia said she knew she was fortunate to have a job allowing her the flexibility to be a caretaker for her parents. Not everyone has the luxury or money to provide all of the care she was able to for her parents, and not all companies allow such flexibility.

The Kidnapping

With the house cleaned out, they decided to bring Margaret back to Minnesota, and Cynthia knew she was supposed to get the court's permission to take her mom out of state. She asked an attorney in Minnesota for advice, but the attorney could not help as their law firm did not have jurisdiction in Missouri. The attorney advised her to inform the local court that they planned to take Margaret out of state. However, Cynthia knew it could take the courts months to respond. Cynthia's take-charge manner kicked in because she knew they could not delay.

The family put their heads together and began to check out nursing homes in Minnesota. Cynthia was hoping to have her mom in a place close to her, but nothing appropriate was available. One of her brothers found a place closer to him and about forty miles from Cynthia. The application was made, and Cynthia began the paperwork transfer from the Missouri nursing home to the new one.

She said, "It was challenging to get all the correct paperwork for both facilities, having the transfer paperwork completed and sent to the new nursing home, and doing this on a tight timeframe. There was almost too much to do in a short amount of time so we could move Mom."

Cynthia met with the staff in the home they chose.

"Will your mom need to be in memory care?" the staff asked her.

"No, she just sits in a chair and does nothing. She does not say any real words. She will not try to leave," Cynthia said with a catch in her voice.

Now, the challenge was getting her mom back home. The drive was too long and flying her on a commercial airplane was a logistical nightmare. Cynthia's brother Mark was a small engine pilot and belonged to a flying club with access to planes. However, his plane was in for repair. He spoke with a pilot friend, who agreed to lend them his plane and even agreed to co-pilot.

Cynthia met her brother Mark at the airport, along with the co-pilot. The propeller started to spin, and they taxied down the runway. It was a beautiful, sunny day as they watched the ground below get smaller.

The flight took five hours. After landing, they rented a car and stopped for lunch. By the time they got to the nursing home, it was later than planned. Cynthia and Mark went in to gather up their mom and her few belongings.

The nursing home would not let them take Margaret until the bill was paid. Cynthia settled with them, and the kidnapping plan was in full force.

"Yes, technically we kidnapped our mom as I should have had permission from the court to move her," Cynthia admitted. "But we just did not have any choice at that point!"

With hope, relief, and apprehension, they settled Margaret on the plane with Cynthia beside her. Margaret was delighted because she loved flying. The first half of the flight went well as she sat looking out of the plane, talking in her own language.

During the last hour of the flight, Margaret had enough–she was tired and wanted out! She repeatedly reached over to open the plane door so she could leave. Cynthia had to keep distracting her, hoping they would land soon without incident.

It was a long final hour.

A New Home

When the plane landed, Susan met them at the airport. The three siblings attempted to convince Margaret to exit the plane, but by the time they arrived, she was exhausted by the journey and wanted to stay in her seat. They coaxed Margaret, and finally, she allowed them to help her out of the plane. They helped Margaret into Cynthia's car as they headed off to the new nursing home with Susan following.

By the time Cynthia and Susan got Margaret settled in her new room, she had rings around her eye, and her face was droopy. Turning down dinner, she crawled into bed. Cynthia went to the office to complete paperwork while Susan sat with their mom until she fell asleep.

Cynthia drove home with barely enough strength to maneuver the car on the roads. Tony had a light dinner waiting, and Cynthia changed clothes, ate, and fell into bed. Tony held her close as she slept soundly for the first time in months.

The nursing home's motto was "A Christ Centered Community." They treated Margaret like family. Cynthia and her siblings were happy and relieved.

"This was a wonderful facility," said Cynthia. "They spent time with Mom. She got a lot of personal attention. The staff was kind, and they paid attention to her. Often, they asked her what she wanted for dinner, even though Mom did not reply. The other residents talked to her."

Cynthia bought her mom new clothes, and she said the staff dressed up her mom like a doll. Margaret had her hair done at Girls and Curls. At first, Cynthia did not like her mom's new hairdo as her hair was brittle and broke off when they set it in curlers. But then she decided, "I don't care what Mom's hair looks like. They are spending time with her, and she is getting a lot of personal attention." Margaret loved it when they combed her hair or massaged her scalp.

Margaret even had a new friend; her name was Gladys. Gladys said, "Margaret is my new best friend!" Cynthia said she would have loved to listen to those "conversations!"

Most of the siblings were able to visit Margaret at the nursing home, although two brothers who lived out of state were not able to make the trip. One sister who lived in the area had not been able to visit her parents when they lived in Missouri, but now, she spent time with her mom on a regular basis. This also helped Cynthia, who had a lot of catching up to do at work and home.

After only two-and-a-half months in her new home, Margaret went swiftly downhill. One morning, Cynthia was called.

"Your mom is not doing well. You need to notify the family to come."

Again, Cynthia felt that heaviness in her chest, remembering hearing those words about her dad.

Cynthia notified her siblings. Margaret laid in bed, unresponsive, with four of her daughters and her oldest granddaughter sitting by her bedside. The hours passed, and later that evening, Margaret peacefully passed on.

Cynthia and her sisters were convinced their father returned for their mother. "My parents were married for fifty-nine years, and they were never far from each other."

Rob and Margaret were laid side by side at the local Veteran's Cemetery where Rob received much-deserved full military honors.

Aftermath

Cynthia's job was not yet done. After her mom died, the remaining assets, which were the house and car, had to go through probate. Cynthia also needed permission from the court in Missouri to sell the assets.

Cynthia found a local realtor in Missouri from a national realty company. It took a while to find a buyer, and once they did, there were more complications with the sale due to the property's layout.

Meanwhile, the buyers wanted to move in before the closing. Cynthia said no, knowing something could go wrong right up to the closing. The potential buyers then asked if they could park their motorhome in the driveway since the local parks were flooded. Cynthia called the local sheriff to ask if the parks were flooded. The sheriff was puzzled and said, "No, there are no floods here." Getting pushback from the realty firm and after having the buyer sign a liability waiver, she finally agreed to the buyer parking their motorhome in the driveway.

The house finally closed, much to Cynthia's relief.

Death and the aftermath can bring out the worst, even in close families. However, Cynthia said, "I have the best siblings. Not one time did any one of the eight question how I was handling our parent's affairs, how the assets were sold, nor how the funds were disbursed. I was upfront and kept everyone informed. No one even argued with how the house was emptied or what we did with all the stuff. I think they were glad it was done. Plus, my parents did not have anything of great value."

All in all, for all of the different personalities and lifestyles, the siblings remain amicable to this day and come through for each other when needed.

Belatedly, Cynthia followed her attorney's advice and reported to the court in Missouri about moving Margaret. She wrapped up the final reports for the state with jurisdiction over her mom. Finally, fifteen months after her mom died, Cynthia was able to divide up the remaining funds among the nine siblings and put this chapter to rest.

But the end of a loved one's life is not the end. Cynthia dealt with retrospection, guilt, and regret after her parents passed. She grieves their loss on this earth, yet she knows Rob and Margaret left their family with an amazing legacy.

Advice

Cynthia, what advice could you give others with aging parents or loved ones who will need care someday?

- You must have a healthcare directive for your loved one, or you could end up having to answer to a court for every decision. I had to send financial reports for every single cent spent on my mom. After she died, it became even more complicated. I had funds that did not need to go through probate due to how they were established and assets that needed to go through probate, namely the house and car. Keeping funds separate so they could be reported properly was challenging. Then add in the estate tax reporting of which I was unfamiliar. (And this coming from a CPA!)

- Also make certain your loved one has a durable power of attorney for financial issues. This is important so that you can handle their finances if they are incapacitated.

- For both of these documents, have an alternative person named. If only one person is named (such as a spouse), and that person becomes incompetent or dies first, other family members will have no ability to act on behalf of the loved one.

- The power of attorney and healthcare directive both become inactive when the person dies. This is why you need a third document: a will. A primary and alternative executor should be named, and both should be able and willing to handle bills, property, and all of the other issues involved with the person's estate.

- If you even remotely think you might need a nursing home for a loved one, do your research ahead of time. Find out the costs. One place we looked at was $10,000 a month. Another one was private care. If the resident runs out of money, they have to leave. You may need a place that has an option to take Medicaid payments.

- Memory care is more difficult to find, especially if a person is prone to wandering or needs a lot of hands-on attention. Check out options specifically for memory care.

- Do your research on care facilities, checking with the regulatory agencies for the quality of the facility and care. You can find a lot of this information on state and federal websites. Does the nursing home have issues that have been identified? Have there been reports of inadequate care? Are there claims filed against the facility? Take a tour and take time to talk with residents. Keep notes about the various places.

- Talk to your parents about finances and get an understanding of their financial situation. Where are their funds located? How much is in each place? Thankfully, my father was willing to talk to me about this. However, there were still a few surprises after he died.

- Most importantly, talk to your parents about end-of-life care and what should be done if they become incapacitated. Anyone listed on the healthcare directive should know their wishes.

Author Reflections

Often, we caretakers think we are prepared for our needs or our loved one's needs as we age. Optimism and denial are adversaries. If someone like Cynthia, who is a CPA and familiar with government regulations, could get caught up in this dreadful situation with her parents, how much more could that happen to any of us?

Preparing for the future may save future stress and heartache, especially in the areas of financial and legal concerns. Cynthia shared this story, hoping to save other families the legal consequences she encountered, which took away from the precious time she had left with her parents.

Chapter 2
To Buddy with Love

"Life must be understood backwards;
but...it must be lived forwards."
– Soren Kierkegarrd

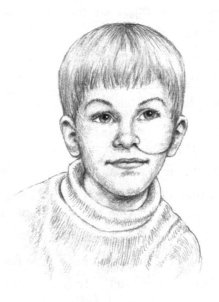

An Unusual Pregnancy

This is the story of an ordinary Minnesota couple who became extra-ordinary parents. Born in a rural area on separate family farms in Minnesota, Landen and Carol learned early they were expected to contribute to the livelihood of the family. There was no advantage to feeling sorry for oneself. Contribute without grumbling or learn the consequences.

Landen worked right alongside his dad on the farm starting at age eight. This was an expectation, and any sign of idleness was at best ignored by his parents and at worse—well, let us just say he learned quickly not to take that route. When Landen turned fifteen, he found a job working on a farm in North Dakota where he continued his education.

Girls were not pampered or allowed to be idle either. Carol helped out wherever she could lend a hand at her home and farm. Again, this was the expectation; families needed everyone to pitch in to survive.

Growing up, they both developed a strong work ethic and were expected to do their best. Landen and Carol grew up to be optimistic people, although they also knew life would not always be easy.

The year was 1968, and life was good. Landen and Carol met, fell in love, married, and moved to an outer suburb of the Twin Cities of Minneapolis and St. Paul, Minnesota. Landen secured a job as a truck driver. Carol enjoyed being a homemaker, and when she got pregnant, they were thrilled. A little red-haired baby girl named Marcie joined the family.

Surprise! When Marcie was only fifteen months old, Carol again realized she was pregnant. Having just been through the pregnancy and birth, they assumed they knew what to expect the second time around. They were looking forward to their second child.

This pregnancy, however, was different.

Quickly, Carol became larger than the first pregnancy. Was she was expecting twins? The doctor did an x-ray to find out because ultrasounds were not used for pregnancies until well into the 1970s. The x-ray showed only one baby and did not reveal any abnormalities.

Carol's due date came and went. She was uncomfortable, and the doctors were concerned about how big she was and what might happen during the birth. They finally decided to induce her, and for the first two days, nothing happened.

Would this baby ever come out? How big would he or she be?

On the third day, Carol went into labor, and they made the short drive to the small, community hospital.

At the hospital, Carol's water broke. There was so much water! The doctor had Carol lay down on the delivery table, and she was told not to move. The doctor tried to slow down the fluid loss. Before long, out came a baby boy born three days before his sister's second birthday.

Indeed, as they feared, things with the baby were not "normal." As part of the initial assessment, the attending nurse listened for his heartbeat. She heard the faint "lub dub" on the right side of his chest instead of the left; his heart was on the opposite side of his body. In addition, he had two thumbs on his right hand.

They named the baby Landen after his dad, but the name "Landen," or "Landen Jr." did not stick long. He was given the nickname "Buddy." His dad decided the little guy earned the nickname "Buddy" after his grandpa, Carol's dad. Landen said, "If he's as strong as his grandpa, he can survive anything!"

"Buddy" stuck with him all his life. When Buddy was enrolled in school, they asked him if he wanted to be called Landen. He emphatically replied, "No, I'm Buddy!"

More problems quickly surfaced in the hospital. Little Buddy tried to suck but had trouble swallowing. At first, they thought it was because he was full of fluid. The next evening, they brought him to Carol with a bottle. By now, Buddy was fussy and hungry. He drank the bottle, but the fluid came right back up. Carol called the nurse, who quickly called the doctor.

The doctor knew something was wrong. He frowned and furrowed his forehead. "This baby needs to get to a hospital with a higher care level." He notified the specialist, and they concluded Buddy would need to be transported the next morning.

It was decided that Landen would drive Buddy to a hospital about twenty-five miles away. Carol wanted to go along, but the doctors told her not to. She was not strong enough to travel. With tears in her eyes, Carol said goodbye to her precious son, not knowing if she would see him again. Her heart was heavy as she curled up in her hospital bed, alone with her thoughts.

Landen and his brother put the hungry baby in the car and started the drive to the larger city hospital. The baby got so quiet and listless during the drive that they thought he was dead. Landen's heart pounded as he pushed down the pedal, not daring to speed too much yet thinking if he did speed, he might get a police escort. He pulled into the hospital with a screech of the tires.

A team was awaiting Buddy's arrival. Dr. T took the baby from Landen and examined him. He discovered Buddy's esophagus did not connect to his stomach; it ended in a pouch at the lung. Immediately, they put the hungry little guy on a feeding tube. Quickly, Buddy's vitals got better, his color returned, and he became more active. The worried dad breathed a sigh of relief and called his wife at the community hospital.

For the next six weeks, they juggled Landen's job, taking care of two-year-old Marcie, and driving to the hospital to spend time with Buddy. They wondered what would happen when Buddy came home.

Before Buddy could go home, Carol had to learn how to care for him. She was given a quick course on tube-feeding. He was fed with a rubber G-tube connected to a glass syringe.

> A gastrostomy tube (also called a G-tube) is inserted through the abdomen, delivering nutrition directly to the stomach. It ensures a person with trouble eating gets the necessary fluid and nutrients.

She also learned to suction fluid out of his mouth so that it would not go into his lungs. This was a constant activity.

The day finally came. Carol said, "I got to bring Buddy home on my birthday!" Life as they knew it would never be "normal" again, but this family created their new normal.

Carol mostly learned how to care for Buddy on her own, applying both instinct and creativity. For example, afraid his taste buds might "die," she dipped the pacifier into the formula and let Buddy suck on it while he was tube fed.

Slowly and constantly, Carol fed Buddy, suctioned his mouth, and fed him again. When she was not caring for Buddy, she was looking after two-year-old Marcie and taking care of the household. Sleep? What was that? Carol barely slept during those first years, other than when Buddy was in the hospital, which was frequent.

Buddy's birth brought a huge financial strain to the family. They did not have health insurance when Buddy was born. When Buddy left the hospital, they owed approximately $4,000. (According to the Bureau of Labor Statistics consumer price index, $4,000 in 1969 is the equivalent to almost $28,000 in 2020.) The icing on the cake was the hospital telling Carol and Landen, "Do not bring your baby back until the bill is paid." What were they to do? All of his specialists practiced at that hospital. Carol said, "None of the other doctors were demanding payment, and here was the big hospital telling us to pay up or not bring our baby back."

They could not even file bankruptcy because the hospital would still close their doors to Buddy if they did not get paid.

Carol and Landen scrambled and were finally able to take out a second mortgage to pay Buddy's hospital bills. It took them five years to pay off the loan. Carol said, "We lived extremely lean because of the medical debt. The anesthesiologists were much more understanding. They would only take what insurance paid. I tried sending them the entire outstanding bill, and they sent the money back. Why couldn't the big hospitals have been more helpful?"

When they finally had health insurance, they were able to stay on track with the medical bills. Carol continued to rely on her analytical mind and creative spirit to keep the family going in lean times.

It was fortunate they were able to take out loans to pay the bills because Buddy had several surgeries to stretch the esophageal tube. They stretched it so much that he was left with a large amount of scar tissue, and it never functioned properly.

As Buddy grew, they discovered other issues. He was deaf in one ear, and he had scoliosis, an s-curve in his spine.

Go! Now!

When Buddy was ten months old, they almost lost him. Landen was a trucker, working nights, and Carol was home alone with the two kids.

Buddy had another ear infection, and he cried and clawed at his ear, not understanding why it hurt. Carol tried to soothe the fussy baby. Finally, when he got sleepy enough, she laid him down. When she went to check on him a short while later, Buddy was barely breathing. Frightened, Carol called the doctor, asking, "I'm trying to keep him breathing. I don't know what to do! Should I meet you at the clinic?"

The doctor said, "No, there isn't time. I'll come to the house."

The doctor came right over and worked on Buddy.

Carol called the neighbor to take care of a frightened Marcie, who said, "This was my earliest memory of life. I was almost three, watching Carol Burnett, and suddenly, the neighbor rushed in to take care of me, while Mom and the doctor raced out with Buddy!"

The doctor drove as fast as he could to the hospital, telling Carol to keep Buddy's head down in the car. He ran into the Emergency Room with Buddy.

The neighbor called Landen's work, who tracked him down on his trucking route.

They sent a tractor out with another driver to finish Landen's run. "Go!" said his coworker as he took over Landen's route. Landen drove the tractor back to the hospital as fast as it would go. He had no idea what he might find when he arrived at the hospital and feared the worst.

He ran in through the emergency room door, searching for his wife and son. They directed him down a long hall. When Landen arrived, he found his wife distraught and Buddy in shock.

Would their baby live?

Scared, Carol and Landen held each other. They could not imagine life without their much-loved son.

Miraculously, Buddy recovered and was able to go home.

Landen was already anxious about the situation with his son. He was worried about how they would pay for Buddy's medical care and how Buddy's special needs would affect the rest of the family. Carol explained, "Buddy's first year was tough. Landen was afraid to love Buddy. He had just lost his mother and was afraid he would lose Buddy too."

Landen's way of coping was to ignore Buddy and pretend he was not there. Carol watched, thinking Landen would come around. She pondered how to motivate her husband to become more involved with Buddy.

Finally, exasperated, Carol told him, "You cannot be this way anymore. I need backing. I cannot take care of Buddy, Marcie, *and you*. You have to love this baby. Whether he lives or not, you have to love him." She threatened to take the two kids and leave him.

In spite of finally having health insurance, money was still scarce, and financial problems added to their household stress. Statistically, the vast majority of couples with a child with a disability end up divorced. The number of couples that split after a child's death is even greater. Could Carol and Landen weather the storm and stay together?

What about Marcie? Would she fade into the background or rebel out of jealousy due to the attention her brother was receiving?

Only time would tell how far this family could expand without shattering.

It is Amazing What a Mom Can Do

In those days, they had few options for outside care. None of their family or friends were willing to care for Buddy as the tube feeding and suctioning made them nervous. Carol's sister was a nurse, and even she was apprehensive.

One night, they were visiting her sister, who lived in a small town two hours away. Her sister agreed to take care of Buddy, and Carol and Landen went out on a dinner date, which was rare.

As Carol's sister fed Buddy, his feeding tube broke. Her sister felt bad but was unable to fix the tube. Normally, when the tube broke, it would be reinserted in Buddy at the local clinic. When Carol and Landen got home, it was late, and no clinic was open. Carol said she would have to take Buddy to the small local hospital.

Her sister said, "That will never work. They do not know you, and it will be an ordeal."

Her sister worked at a nursing home, so she went and got a catheter and tubes. Carol replaced Buddy's broken tube herself.

Later, she told Buddy's doctor about her "fix-it" session. The doctor was impressed and said Carol could do the repair all of the time. So, she did.

"When it's your child, it's amazing what you can do," commented Carol.

Eventually, when she took Buddy to the doctor, Carol was the doctor's assistant. They had to dilate his esophagus to allow him to eat through his mouth. The doctor would put the dilator in Buddy's stomach and pull it through his mouth. Carol resolutely held his legs and arms down and talked soothingly to her baby boy.

Eventually, Carol learned to dilate him at home. "I'd push the dilator down his throat and be a mean mom and dilate him. I closed my eyes and went into my other world," she said with a shudder.

The strings used to dilate his esophagus were left coming out of his nose and mouth. People would ask Carol, "Why does he have strings in his nose and mouth?"

Carol knew people were curious, but it was hard to "hear" her son was "different." She said, "My response all depended on how they asked. Some people genuinely cared, and I would be honest with them about Buddy's condition. But if they asked sarcastically or in a negative way, I would respond, 'I pull one string and he walks; I pull the other string and he talks.'"

Even then, Carol took the opportunity to educate people about her precious Buddy. Plus, she kept her sense of humor.

Little sister Marcie did not understand why people would ask; Buddy's condition was normal to her. She proudly showed me pictures on the family wall of Buddy and her with the strings in his nose. They were approximately three and five, huddled together in a typical brother-sister pose.

When Buddy got older, he would say, "Feed me. Hungry." Carol made runny cereal and kept it on his taste buds even while he was tube fed. He ate like that until he was five years old. By then, they hoped he would be able to eat food through his mouth at school. The medical team decided he could handle esophageal surgery, so they cut the esophagus in half, split it in two, and stitched him up. After that, he learned to eat.

I made the mistake of asking Carol if she was able to work (meaning work outside the home). I got the "mom" look! "Did I work? I worked constantly for years. I barely slept!"

She also reminded me there were no daycares back then for special needs kids, and even if there had been a daycare option, they could not afford it. Also, who would be willing to take care of Buddy and all his needs?

To compensate, Landen worked up to eighty hours a week driving a truck. They always had medical bills to pay. People asked them why they did not put money away for retirement, and Carol responded, "We did not have any extra money for retirement. I would retire when I knew my son was taken care of. What happens to me would not matter."

As Buddy got older, Landen slowly overcame his apprehension and learned to interact with Buddy. In truth, Landen loved Buddy so much it hurt, and he was frightened he would lose his son. I asked if Landen and Buddy were close when Buddy got older, and Carol said, "Oh, yes. They were very close."

School Days

Carol and Landen worried about what would happen when Buddy started school. Would he be able to learn? How would the school handle a child with special needs?

Buddy was a summer baby, so between his late birthday and his medical needs, Carol and Landen waited until he was six to enroll him in school.

Due to the string he previously had in his nose and mouth, Buddy had developed a "lazy tongue." He had speech therapy before he started school and during school. He was able to eat, although slowly.

Carol introduced Buddy to his teachers in person, and she gave them a list of instructions:

- Have Buddy sit on the teacher's right so he can hear.
- Seat him in the front of the room.
- When it comes to lunch, Buddy knows what he is able to eat.
- If he jumps up from the table and runs to the bathroom, let him go; it means he has to clear out the food pouch.
- If he asks for another milk or water, give it to him.

When Buddy almost died at ten months old, they believed he had a brain injury, which became apparent when he started school. Buddy learned differently, but as was the custom, he was mainstreamed in the public school with both regular classes and special education classes. A team of special ed teachers worked with Buddy too, and some of them he had for three years.

When Buddy could hear what was being read, it increased his comprehension. The teacher read out loud to him in a separate room, or he would sit in the corner and read out loud to himself.

Buddy was friendly and outgoing. He was a kid who was loved by his teachers. While in middle school, he was often selected to bring the attendance record to the administrative office where he would stop and chat with the office staff. One day on the way back to his regular classroom he bopped into an open door, where Mr. Jones was preparing for his English class the next hour. They struck up a conversation, and Mr. Jones recognized Buddy's inquisitive nature. He arranged to spend extra time with Buddy, and together they read stories such as *The Adventures of Huckleberry Finn*. Later, when the class got quizzed on the book, Buddy already knew all of the answers.

On the other hand, Buddy frustrated his mom. He would not sit down and do his schoolwork like he should, or he purposely left his homework at school. In spite of having learning problems, Buddy was quick and witty. He could talk his way out of any situation with his teachers but not his mom!

When Buddy was in seventh grade, the teachers enhanced his learning through specialized auditory teaching. When it was time to take tests, the special ed teacher read the questions out loud to him, and he would answer. The special ed staff worked diligently with him, and he was able to graduate from high school.

Marcie was on the other end of the spectrum; she was a gifted child who learned quickly. Her parents had to search for ways to keep her challenged. Carol said, "We were blessed to be in our school district. Both of our kids were able to succeed."

Carol and Landen never treated Buddy like he was handicapped. Chores around the house were expected to be done by both Marcie and Buddy. They were raised to behave and be respectful. Other than the couple of restrictions on physical activities, Buddy was a "regular boy." He rode his bike, drove snowmobiles when he got older, and played non-contact games.

Marcie and Buddy were a normal brother and sister. They played together, and they fought. Marcie was his biggest defender; she would beat up other children who picked on Buddy. (Buddy did not necessarily appreciate having his big sister coming to his rescue though.)

"He was just my little brother," explained Marcie. "He loved scaring me! I hated to ride behind him on the snowmobile because he would deliberately try to frighten me. We were like peanut butter and jelly, but Buddy was a different type of jelly."

Marcie's friends would ask why Buddy's shoulders were crooked. Marcie said this question always surprised her because she did not notice. The surgeons advised they could straighten out his shoulders, but there was a five percent chance of paralysis. His parents chose not to take that chance.

Growing Up Fearless and Friendly

Buddy completed eighth grade, the last year before entering high school. The school held a graduation, proudly attended by Carol, Landen, and Marcie. The highlight of completing eighth grade was a class trip to a local amusement park the week after graduation. Unfortunately, Buddy also needed spine fusion surgery that summer. They knew he would be in a body cast for three months, so the surgery was scheduled as soon as school was out.

When Carol learned about the class trip she asked, "Should we reschedule the surgery, Buddy?"

Buddy said, "Mom, let's get it done. I don't want to be in a body cast next school year."

Another surgery, another hospital stay, and more recovery. Again, they did not know how Buddy would react to this new surgery.

"I should not have worried," reported Carol. They barely got Buddy home from the hospital, and he was out riding his bike in his body cast. His sense of balance was off, but he quickly figured out how to compensate. His mom remembered, "You just couldn't slow this kid down."

I asked her if she had anxiety, remembering when my sons took off on their bikes the first time. "No, I did not. I just went with it."

After Buddy's spine was fused, there were a couple of off-limits activities. He could not play contact sports such as football or soccer, and he could not jump head-first into the water. Fortunately, those activities did not interest him, so it was not a problem.

Buddy was in Boy Scouts, and Landen was his scout leader. The summer of his spine surgery was the year the troop was to go canoeing at the Boundary Waters. Landen was worried Buddy might drown in his body cast, but Carol said he would do fine. He knew his limits, and he had survived this far! As predicted, Buddy had a great time, and Landen and Buddy grew even closer.

Buddy drove motorbikes when he was little and snowmobiles when he was older. Carol and Landen did not talk about how to raise Buddy, and they did not have a discussion on treating him like any other kid. They just did it. They were raised to work hard and put their whole hearts into whatever tasks they had to take on, so their children were naturally raised the same way.

"Besides, if we told him he was not able to ride a bike, he would have done it anyway. If we told him not to go over bumps, he would have gone over bigger bumps. 'Poor Buddy' was never in our language," exclaimed Carol.

The doctors wanted to see Buddy when he turned eighteen. They asked him, "What do you like to do for fun?"

Buddy said, "I motorcycle."

The doctor was shocked at how active and fearless Buddy had become.

Marcie said about her brother, "Buddy and I were always expected to contribute, to always do our best. I had a paper route until I was sixteen, then Buddy took it over. It took him forever to do the route because he was too busy chatting with people."

Buddy's friendly nature lit up the world for everyone he met. While many teenagers do not have time for adults, he knew all of the neighbors and talked with them on a regular basis.

When Buddy was sixteen, he got an after-school job working at a service station. He cleaned the building, pumped gas, and washed windows, smiling and chatting with the customers.

Henry, the owner of the gas station, was one of Buddy's best teachers. Once, Buddy accidentally brought money home. The next morning, he took it out of his pocket and gave it to Henry.

Instead of questioning Buddy, Henry thanked him and taught him how to balance the register right down to the penny.

Once in a while, Buddy would forget to lock the doors at the station. Henry would call him, and instead of lecturing Buddy, Henry insisted he get out of bed, go in, and lock the doors. Buddy learned so much from Henry, who loved Buddy like a son. Other kids would steal but not Buddy. He adored that job. He did it from when he was sixteen until he was twenty-one.

Adulthood

Buddy attended a technical school after he graduated from high school. He studied to be a diesel mechanic but decided that was not for him. He did not want to be cooped up inside. He wanted to drive a truck like his dad.

Landen said he would teach Buddy how to drive. Landen's company was willing to hire Buddy but not yet. Buddy was only twenty-one, and to drive, he needed to be twenty-three. Landen threatened to quit if they would not take Buddy on. The company wanted to keep Landen, so they let him teach Buddy how to drive.

Landen was so sad the day Buddy said, "Dad, I want my own truck." He missed the camaraderie of driving with his son and even missed their "arguments."

Buddy fulfilled his dream, bought a truck, and became a truck driver. He drove back and forth across the country. His family was surprised because he could not move his neck well to see in all of the truck's mirrors, but Buddy compensated. And of course, nothing ever stopped Buddy! He loved driving a truck so much. During one especially bad winter up north, he took a job driving between California and Texas just so he could stay on the road.

When he was home, Buddy was a great neighbor. He would grab a couple of beers and visit with his elderly neighbors. He could talk to anybody.

In his early thirties, Buddy fell in love with Kim. They got married, and Buddy adopted Kim's two children. They loved to ride Buddy's Harley. Because Kim was short, she could not manage her own bike, so she rode with him. They made a wonderful life together.

> Tragically, in 2009 at age thirty-nine, Buddy died in a trucking accident. His heartbroken family was crushed.

The Good-bye

Many of Buddy's teachers, school buddies, and Boy Scout friends came to his funeral along with their parents. On his obituary page, his friends wrote:

"I went to school with Buddy and have always thought of him fondly. He was a decent, kind & genuine person whose uplifting outlook on life was a true pleasure to be around."

"Buddy…touched many lives…I know Buddy knew he was loved by many and missed by so many…Thank YOU Buddy for sharing your life with us!!"

"I will miss my friend, a person you could call at any time you needed help. Thank you for all the great memories. I can't say it enough: 'I WILL MISS MY FRIEND…' I thank you

Landen and Carol for your loving, kind, good-spirited son. Only Buddy could make anyone, anywhere feel included."

"I will always remember Buddy with that devilish twinkle in his eye, and a smile that always kept you guessing. Our sympathy goes out to Buddy's family. He will be greatly missed."

Advice

Carol, what advice do you have for people with children with challenges?

- Do not unnecessarily limit them or coddle them; let them be kids. Buddy could go and match any kid for dirt. You have to encourage them.
- Be strong; they have to learn how to live life.
- Stop and look at your kid and say, "Is there is a reason why he or she cannot do something?"
- Your child will have to leave home someday. They have to learn to live life and take care of themselves as much as possible.
- Educate the schools and teachers. Be your child's advocate.
- You also need to advocate for your child with the medical community. This includes keeping track of medical records, medications, and educating medical professionals, especially if your child has an unusual situation.

What made you so resilient?

Buddy made us resilient. He would not allow himself to be babied or be told he was different from other kids. As time went on, Landen and I supported each other—and we stayed together!

How did you help Marcie deal with her brother?

Marcie never felt left out. Our family had a warped sense of normal. When Buddy went to the hospital, Marcie also went along. The hospital had a fantastic play area, and she helped the other kids play with play dough and other toys.

One time, there was a little girl from another state in the hospital. The play lady said to Marcie, "Oh I'm glad you're here. This little girl needs someone to play with." Marcie went and played with the little girl. The girl's mother was so happy, she said that was just what her daughter needed.

We did not make a conscious decision to include Marcie. That was just how it was. We did know we needed to give Marcie something special though. That was when her daddy took her to Mr. Donut.

What helped you cope? Friends, faith, anything else?

At first, the only thing that helped was sleep. I slept when Buddy was in the hospital. Otherwise, it was 24/7 caretaking. Faith came later, and it evolved with time. I believe the Lord only gives you what you can handle.

Our support system was friends and neighbors. They helped with Marcie. We had two friends who were always there for us, and they brought meals. Our family always lent a hand and a listening ear.

Marcie, how did you cope?

I had a different kind of resilience. The only outings I knew were trips to the hospital. I remember sitting in the waiting area alone, a little girl about three or four years old under the watchful eye of a little old lady at the information desk. Meanwhile, my parents checked Buddy in for one of his many stays.

Back then, children were not allowed on the floor of hospitals. So, I sat in a chair alone, waiting for my parents to return and pick me up.

Most of the time, my mom stayed with Buddy, and Dad picked me up and took me to the donut shop for a treat. We did not go out to eat. Buddy could not eat regular food, plus he regurgitated. So, going out for a donut with Dad was a special treat.

Because Buddy saw a number of different specialists, we often spent time at different hospitals for his follow-up exams or procedures. I knew which hospitals had the best playrooms. Finally, a children's hospital was built, and Buddy was one of the first patients.

In second grade "Show and Tell," I shared how I got to eat at McDonald's the night before. My class could not understand why that was such a treat because "everyone goes to McDonald's." The teacher, who knew about Buddy's situation, talked about how our family cared for my special brother.

We had a normal life. We went camping and hung out with cousins. I never felt like Buddy got special attention, and I was never excluded.

Marcie, did your family ever learn the name of Buddy's disabilities?

I always loved science, and my background is in biology and genetics. The doctors had explained how Buddy's condition just happened in pregnancy; they did not believe it was genetic. One time in school, I ran across a description for "Vater Syndrome." I asked the professor if Buddy could have "Vater Syndrome." The professor said it was likely. That alone explained a lot about my brother.

Vater Syndrome is a term used when a child is diagnosed with birth defects in three or more body parts. These birth defects are not genetic. They happen in pregnancy for unknown reasons.

Author Reflections

The tragedy is not that Buddy was born with a variety of birth defects. Through caring for Buddy, his parents learned a love beyond anything they could have imagined. Buddy will always live in their hearts.

Nor is the tragedy about Marcie, even though she missed out on many "normal" childhood experiences. As Marcie grew up and approached adulthood, she developed empathy for anyone experiencing discrimination. She speaks up not only for those having physical or developmental differences, but for all people who may be belittled, regardless of race, religion, lifestyle, or social class.

The true tragedy is that Buddy was taken from his loved ones too soon.

Chapter 3
Life on Hold

"But if a widow has children or grandchildren, these should learn first of all to put their religion into practice by caring for their own family and so repaying their parents and grandparents, for this is pleasing to God."
– 1 Timothy 5:4

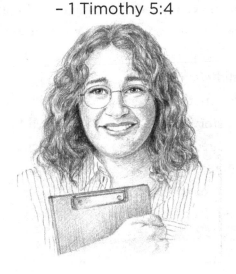

Introduction

If I asked you to put your life, your dreams, and your plans on hold for an unknown amount of time, would you be willing?

By the way, this will be one of the most difficult seasons of your life. It will result in you crying in a crumpled heap in a public restroom.

You might say, "No, thank you!"

And then I say, "Friend, it is to care for a loved one. If you do not step up, he or she may spend the last years of his or her life in an institution, cared for by strangers."

Your "no" might change to a "maybe." Still, many of us would hesitate, and more of us could not even consider this as an option. Perhaps you work, or you have a full house. Maybe you have a disability yourself and cannot care for another person. Or maybe your loved one just needs more nursing care than you are able to provide.

What would have to come into alignment for a family to care for a loved one in their home? What if you know in your heart this is a calling? Life experiences have prepared you for this moment!

What would you do?

My friends Sandra and Ken were faced with this very question.

This is the story of Joe, a man who loved life and loved his family. As Joe aged, he began to have problems caring for himself and his home.

Sandra, Joe's daughter, loves people. She is a compassionate and loyal friend. Her husband, Ken, is patient and thoughtful, a man who looks to God for strength.

While Sandra and Ken did not know how long Joe could stay in their home or if they would be up to the task, they readily said, "Yes, Dad can come live with us." This is their caretaking story.

Joe

As a young man, Joe answered the call to ministry. After attending seminary, he married the love of his life, Elaine. As a minister, Joe shepherded several congregations in the upper Midwest of the United States while Elaine shared her musical and teaching talents with the parishioners. Elaine loved to hear about their lives and ministered in her own way. Joe and Elaine had four children, a son and three daughters, within eight years.

Being in the ministry was not always easy, especially for Joe and Elaine's kids. In those days, they moved ministers around, not wanting them to get too attached to one church. It was hard to put down roots, and usually, money was scarce.

People could be critical, which they found to be true in some small towns. Perhaps they did not realize how words cut into tender hearts. Sandra, their oldest daughter, would revert to those hurt feelings when criticized later in her life.

Joe was by nature reserved, but he was able to reach into the hearts of those he ministered to with a compassionate and genuine nature. Later in life, Joe worked at a nonprofit serving the homeless and rebuilding lives one by one. As a Christian, Joe lived his beliefs. His best day was when he could serve others.

Elaine had a heart for the elderly and people with disabilities. She worked in a nursing home for a short period of time. She willingly took both Joe's parents and her parents into their home when they were older and needed more care. Later, Elaine did in-home foster care for people with disabilities. She was a loving example of how to care for and have fun with older adults. Like their mom, two of her daughters worked in care homes, and Elaine's example set the stage for her husband's care many years later.

Sadly, cancer overcame Elaine, and she died in her early sixties. The loss was heartbreaking for Joe as they were a true husband and wife team. Following her death, Joe lived alone in their big house, tended his garden, and cared for the yard. He expected to live in his house until God called him home.

Joe enjoyed his family, spending time helping his son and daughters with projects, and spending time with the grandkids. He played games with them and easily demonstrated God's love through his servanthood. Joe was also intelligent and analytical. At his funeral, Joe's youngest daughter described their many conversations about the meaning of God and life as "iron sharpens iron."

Joe was an orderly person, and as he aged, the daily patterns of his life became more important. He demonstrated a common trait of the aging: comfort zones shrink as we contend with physical, emotional, and brain changes.

Joe ate the same food for breakfast, lunch, and dinner, set the table the same way, and went to bed at the same time every night. Household chores had to be done in a particular way. Living alone for over twenty years only reinforced these patterns in Joe.

If there was something Joe did not like, he did not hesitate to let a family member know how he felt. He liked to give advice, although he did so in a gentle manner. For example, Joe would quietly watch one of his kids struggle with assembling an item. When it finally came together, Joe would point out,

"That is the right way to do it!" Or he might come out with, "A smart thing to say," when someone reached a conclusion that echoed his viewpoint.

Joe liked getting Christmas and birthday gifts from the kids, and when he got something he liked, you could tell. The family caught on, and one year, one of his daughters gave him seven gifts, knowing the first six were silly and useless. Joe just nodded as he opened each gift. He got to the seventh gift, expecting another can of soup or a pen. He broke out in a big smile when the gift was a hat he had been admiring. "I like this hat!" Everyone chuckled, including Joe.

Joe also relished baked goods. The family knew they could not go wrong with a sweet roll or brownie for their dad.

Sandra

Sandra is a mixture of her mom's bubbly personality and her dad's intensity. She loves people, from the youngest child to the oldest senior. When she bursts out laughing, you cannot help but laugh with her. Sandra is compassionate, describing herself as "having a lot of grace for people."

Like her dad, Sandra likes structure and order. She ran an in-home daycare for twenty-eight years where children thrived under her consistent care.

Family is everything to her. As the oldest of the four siblings, Sandra is loving, loyal, and the one to keep the family in touch.

But even for a person like Sandra, whose love for family is steady and fast, a person can be stretched almost to the breaking point. She would find out how far love could bend without breaking, like the willow tree in a spring storm.

In the early 1970s, the world was in a recession. Sandra's parents had few financial resources, and she knew she would need a skill to help with upcoming college expenses. She took classes and became a Certified Nursing Assistant (CNA). Sandra did an internship in a clinic where she learned the basics of care. When it was time to get a job, Sandra knew right away she wanted to work with the elderly. She found a job in the local nursing home.

A CNA provides hands-on healthcare to patients, helping with bathing, dressing, and attending to the basic activities of life. A CNA takes vital signs such as temperature or blood pressure and looks for bruises, skin tears, or signs of illness. One of the most important skills a CNA learns is how to safely transport patients, moving them in and out of bed and turning them or transitioning them to toileting without hurting the patient or the caregiver.

In college, Sandra relied on her training, working in two different nursing homes. The first one was a long walk from the college in an unsafe neighborhood in the midst of the city. Sandra looked for new employment, finding a job in a care home right next to campus. This home was a much better fit for her.

Nothing suited her better than laughing with the residents while she cared for their needs.

What Sandra did not know was how this job would prepare her for one of the most important tasks of her life. An undertaking that would stretch her physically, emotionally, and spiritually. A task that would become a mission, bringing smiles and tears.

Ken

Tall with dark hair and a big smile, Ken is one of those guys you cannot help but like. He is easygoing, loving, and accepting. His steadfast nature was formed where he grew up in a close-knit family in the southwestern United States.

His mom was a missionary overseas who got caught up in World War II. When she returned to the U.S., she met Ken's dad, who was blind since birth. Together, they ministered to the blind, becoming domestic missionaries. They had three children, two daughters and a son.

During the summer, Ken's parents sent the children to their uncle and aunt's house so the kids could spend time with their uncle. They felt it was important they be around a man who could interact with them using his sight. Their aunt and uncle were a second family.

Ken's parents brought up their three children to be honest, hardworking, and serve God. Ken felt like he had to become a missionary as many of his family had done. He attended a Bible College in the Midwest where he first majored in Bible studies and missions. But Ken eventually discerned he did not have the calling to be a missionary. He sought career counseling where he realized computer programming was a much better fit for him. Ken was happy in his chosen profession and was still able to serve his church and family as a Christian man.

Family

Sandra also attended the same Bible college. In those days, if a person did not have a home church, the college assigned a local place of worship to be their "Christian Service Station." Ken was assigned a suburban church where he could serve. Sandra chose the same church as she had family who were regular attendees. As Ken had a car and Sandra did not, he routinely gave her a ride to church.

The two clicked early on and knew they were meant for each other. After marrying, they bought a 1,400 square foot rambler with four bedrooms. They settled in the suburban neighborhood of their home church and joyfully welcomed three daughters. Sandra loved running her in-home daycare and loving on the little ones while she cared for her own daughters. Ken continued as a computer programmer for a local corporation and served on different committees and boards at their local church.

Ken and Sandra were always ready to share their resources and home with others. Several of Sandra's younger siblings lived with them from time to time. A good friend of Sandra's who was a single parent got quite ill one summer, and Sandra invited her nine-year-old daughter to stay with them while her friend recovered. The girl was also a good friend of Sandra's middle daughter, and she is part of their family to this day.

I asked Sandra if there was anything about their marriage that was difficult. Sandra said she would get frustrated with Ken when she asked him to do a task around the house and he "did not have time." But if someone from church would call and ask him for help, he was right there to assist! Like Sandra's dad, Ken loved to serve others.

There were ups and downs in life, like in any family, but their marriage was strong, and they raised their children with love.

Parkinson's Disease

In 2011, Joe was diagnosed with Parkinson's Disease.

> Parkinson's affects nerve cells in the brain responsible for body movement. Patients show symptoms such as tremors, slowness, stiffness, and balance problems. There is no cure for Parkinson's Disease. However, there are a variety of medications used to treat symptoms.

Joe did fairly well for the next three years, but in his mid-eighties, the symptoms became more severe. Joe's hands would shake, and he had a couple of falls in the house. His son Jerry, who lived the nearest to Joe, came over to help with yard work, grocery shopping, and putting on his dad's knee-length compression socks. Jerry and his wife faithfully took Joe to church with them, which was a social outlet for Joe. Jerry's two children were blessed to be able to spend more time with their grandpa.

But Joe went slowly downhill. They discovered he was getting up three or four times a night to go to the bathroom and was using his dresser to pull himself up. It was becoming clear that Joe needed more care, but he insisted, "I'm fine. I can manage by myself."

Falls

> The Centers for Disease Control (CDC) says that each year, millions of people sixty-five and older fall. More than one out of four older people fall each year and falling once doubles your chances of falling again. While some falls do not cause injury, many falls result in broken bones, including hip fractures or head injury.

Joe's odds of falling were high, and sure enough, one day, he fell outside. After Joe landed and caught his breath, he realized he had fallen behind his car. Any view of Joe from the road was blocked. Joe tried to push himself up, but he could not propel himself off the ground. He was stuck, hurt, and scared.

Fortunately, a neighbor eventually came outside and helped Joe up. They called Jerry, who took his dad in to the doctor to get checked out.

Joe was told part of the reason he was falling was because he was dehydrated. Joe had good intentions but would get busy around the house and forget to drink his water. He became uncertain and afraid to go out.

Not long after the outside fall, Joe was alone in his house and had a more serious fall. He managed to call the emergency number, 911, and the ambulance came to take Joe to the hospital. When Jerry and his family heard, they experienced that stabbing fear in the pit of their stomachs as they headed to the hospital to see what happened to their dad this time.

The family had new causes for fear and anxiety, followed by a long wait for treatment. This time, Joe was hospitalized for several days, and then he was sent to a nursing home for rehabilitation. Joe was not happy in the nursing home; he was lonely and scared.

After he went home, Jerry started spending the night with his dad, which was difficult as he worked full time. This was clearly not a long-term solution.

At that point, the family had to face the facts: Joe could no longer live alone.

What to Do About Dad

The family discussed what to do. The two younger daughters were not in situations where they could take their dad in, and Jerry and his wife still had two children at home. His wife homeschooled and was a major contributor to a homeschooling coop. They were willing to take in their dad, but it would have presented challenges.

Sandra always thought she would take care of her parents as they aged. She had admired how her mom took care of her older relatives and others, and Sandra wanted to provide that type of care for her parents. Unfortunately, her mom died before Sandra could take care of her, but when it became clear her dad needed more care, Sandra and Ken were faced with a decision.

Sandra knew her dad would be miserable in a nursing home. Because of Sandra's prior CNA nursing home experience, she knew the basics of caring for a fragile adult. She was willing to move her dad into their home but needed to discuss it with Ken.

Sandra stated, "After prayer and searching his own heart and wanting to be supportive of me, Ken agreed Dad could move in our home." Ken knew Sandra could not take on the task alone, and he agreed to partner with Sandra in "Dad's" care, as he called his father-in-law.

They knew they were in a good place in life to take on this new task. Sandra and Ken felt like God had prepared them for this time, and it was the right decision. So, in 2014, Joe's house was put up for sale. The family took on the task of cleaning out the house where Joe had lived for over thirty-five years. Joe came out of the nursing home and moved into Ken and Sandra's home.

Did they have time to thoroughly think through the ramifications of this decision? Was their house prepared for a fragile senior? Were they the only two in the house, and was Sandra fully retired from daycare? No. But are any of us completely prepared when a family crisis stares us in the face?

Physical and occupational therapists came into the house where they both evaluated Joe and provided suggestions on how to modify the house. Sandra and Ken ordered the equipment Joe would need to live in his new environment. The physical therapist told Sandra she may be able to take care of her dad for a year.

Was that to be the case? Would his Parkinson's disease progress at a pace where they could no longer care for him at home? Would exhaustion and stress overwhelm Sandra and Ken? These were big unknowns.

If you could meet Sandra, you would discover she loves a challenge. And if you knew Ken, you would know he not only said it was okay for Dad to move in but also was committed to the success of the new arrangement. But would good intentions be enough?

Dad Moves In

The new normal began. Like many choices we make, caring for an aging parent is a major life-changing experience. Sandra now acknowledges it was a much bigger job than they expected, and it stretched Sandra and Ken beyond what they thought was possible. It affected their home life, their marriage, their family connections, and their relationship with Sandra's dad in ways they could not imagine. Through it, they drew strength from each other and experienced the grace and comfort of God.

Joe had lived by himself since his wife died in 1998, and he was used to doing things a certain way. Sandra can laugh at this now, but it was not so funny back in the day. When he first came to live with them, he was particular about how he wanted things done. For example, he wanted his flatware by his plate in a certain order, as he had done at home.

Midwesterners are known for their indirect way of communication. Joe would say, "I don't have a spoon." His daughter understood this language and would promptly get him the spoon.

Ken, who had grown up in another part of the country, never got used to this indirect communication method. He would say, "Dad, do you want a spoon?" encouraging Joe to ask outright for what he needed. Ken, patient though he was, remained puzzled by Joe's inability to come right out and ask for what he needed.

Sandra initially catered to her dad in every way. This became exhausting. Finally, she let her dad know he would have to try harder to adapt to their household, even if it was not exactly how he was used to living.

Still, Joe liked his schedule. He was always asking Sandra, "What's next?" If she overlooked or skipped one of the daily activities, Joe would notice and ask, "Are we going to exercise today?" or "Isn't it time for me to read in my chair?" Joe liked his life to be orderly.

Sandra said the first year was the hardest. In addition to getting used to another member in the household, there were other stressors. Sandra was still caring for two school-aged daycare kids. Both children were from split homes and had their own issues. They were also likely acting out as a reaction to Sandra's shared attention between her daycare and her dad. Sandra and the parents eventually agreed the kids were getting older and could move on to other levels of care.

After twenty-eight years in daycare, Sandra gave up her beloved profession as a daycare provider. It was a bittersweet end. She had loved and cared for so many children, yet now she was called to provide caregiving in a different way.

From time to time, Ken and Sandra opened their home to others in need of housing. During this same time, two other family members lived in the household. Sandra's niece Maggie had moved in with her young son about a year before Joe came. It was meant to be a short-term situation, but they ended up staying three years.

Before Joe moved in, they all did a fairly good job of giving each other space, but everything was magnified when Joe became a resident. Maggie was afraid Sandra and Ken would make her move out, but Ken and Sandra made a room in the basement for her and her son. The niece was upset her beloved grandpa was failing in health, and he was not always the cheerful, game-playing grandpa she had grown up knowing.

Space became a premium, especially during mealtimes. It was an adjustment, and at times, tearful for all.

Goals

When Joe moved in, Sandra asked him about his goals and what was most important to him. Joe's response was the following things:

- He did not want to be in pain.
- No nursing homes!
- He wanted more time to read.

Two components were crucial for Joe to stay pain-free and out of the nursing home. The first was exercise. He would do exercises specific for Parkinson's patients, and he would slowly walk on the treadmill for fifteen minutes at a time. Sandra would play hymns for him while he walked, and often when she came in the room, her dad had tears in his eyes.

As time went on, Joe's use of the treadmill became five minutes or less, and then it became too dangerous.

Instead, they would have Joe take regular walks around the house. He could do it by himself at first, but later they placed a sturdy safety belt around his waist, holding it as he walked to add stability.

The second critical component was keeping Joe hydrated. Sandra said this was the most difficult part of caregiving on an on-going basis. They quickly realized Joe did not want to drink much water during the day because it meant he would have to get up and use the restroom during the night. They consulted a doctor who explained to Joe that he had to drink more water during the day to flush out his kidneys. If he did not drink water, he would still have to go to the bathroom at night, but it would make him ill. Joe said he understood, but he still had to be reminded to drink water.

Joe liked tea and "Postum," a powdered roasted-grain beverage substituted for coffee. The doctors said coffee was not good for Joe because it interfered with some of his medications. He also enjoyed juice with his breakfast. All helped with his hydration.

Joe's third goal, being able to read, became more difficult for him. Sandra or other family members would read to him. Sometimes, Joe would choose to lay back in his elevated chair to listen to tapes, which gave Sandra more time to take care of the house and his other needs. Joe especially liked to listen to the Bible on CDs, it gave him comfort and brought back memories of the years he was in ministry.

Progression and Loss

Sandra's siblings pitched in as much as possible. Sandra and Ken tried to get help on Friday nights so they could have a date night. They recognized it was important to keep their marriage strong and to have time to communicate in private.

At times, Sandra and Ken's adult children, who all lived in different states, would come home to care for their grandpa so Sandra and Ken could get away.

During the first year, Jerry and his family came and picked up Joe for church, allowing Sandra and Ken to attend their own worship services. But eventually, it became too hard for Joe to stand up in church, and they all agreed Joe could no longer attend the beloved church where he and his wife had worshiped for many years. Aging and disability often results in one sad loss after another.

Sandra's one outlet giving her joy was teaching Sunday School. At first, Ken would stay home while Sandra taught Sunday School, after which she would come home to be with her dad while Ken went to church. This was not a long-term solution because church was not only their spiritual home but also where they had many friends and social activities.

Parkinson's continued to take its toll on Joe. While it manifests itself differently in individuals, common symptoms include the following:

- Changes in speaking, voice may drop.
- Shuffling or "freezing" when a person first starts to walk or changes direction.
- Trouble swallowing.
- Falling.
- Problems with balance and coordination.
- Slower movements.

Joe experienced most of these, other than the speaking problems, which was a blessing. Though occasionally, he had difficulty smiling.

Joe was having trouble with balance and standing. One example was his desire to stand up and use the toilet as he had done all his life. Usually, Sandra helped her dad up out of bed, but one day, Joe decided he wanted to give Sandra a "gift" of a good night's sleep, so he got up to go the bathroom alone. She suddenly woke up at 4:00 a.m. and jumped out of bed to check on her dad. She could see he had gone to the bathroom on his own and reminded him again not to get up alone.

Joe agreed, but sometimes, he "forgot" to ask for help. He carefully balanced himself until one time he fell backward. Sandra came running into the bathroom and saw her dad had fallen. She helped him up.

Joe was already having shoulder and hip pain, and the fall exaggerated his pain. A couple of days later, Sandra took him to the doctor. Although the fall added to his pain, the doctor was unable to isolate the original source of the aching shoulders and hip.

"Could Dad have cortisone shots?" Sandra asked.

The family doctor referred Joe to a specialist. Sandra took her dad to the specialist and advocated again for him to receive cortisone shots. The specialist agreed, and Joe was prescribed periodic shots. Once a month Sandra drove her dad to other side of the city in freeway traffic. Sandra laughs at the time her dad told her, "You are a good driver in traffic." Having learned to drive in a small town, Sandra says it was the only time in her life someone told her she was a good driver!

As her dad's caregiver, Sandra knew that she would need to be an advocate for her dad. She worked to articulate his issues when he could not do so himself, and she found it helpful to bring notes and written questions to doctor's appointments.

Help on Board

Lack of sleep is a common problem for caregivers. Joe wanted Sandra to tuck him in at night and have his mouth sprayed with a moisturizing liquid. The nighttime routine was initially comforting for both Joe and Sandra. But then Joe started to believe he needed Sandra's help more often, and he would call for her during the night to have his mouth moistened.

Sandra said, "Dad, only call for us when you need help getting up for the bathroom." Joe agreed, and feeling bad, he would try to get up and use the commode, which was now next to his bed, by himself.

For a while, this was a success. Until it was not.

Joe fell getting to the commode.

Sandra reflected on the difference between running a daycare and caring for an aging parent. When she ran her daycare, she would feed the children when needed, help them go potty, and tuck them in for naps. They grew more independent as time went on. When caring for her elderly dad, he became more dependent. It is draining on all when abilities start to fade away.

Sandra no longer let him go on the commode during the night. She set the nursery monitor to alert her and Ken every few hours so one of them could get up with him.

At first, Sandra and Ken took turns getting up with Joe. Ken would get up every other time, even though he was working full time. The lack of sleep was wearing on him. They tried having Sandra get up with Joe the first four times, then Ken would get up at four a.m. and help Dad. That even got too exhausting for Ken, so he would get up with Joe at five a.m., leaving most of the nighttime duties to Sandra.

Sandra says Ken was the biggest supporter. He was kind and firm with his father-in-law, pitching in whenever possible, but Ken needed to work and be alert at his job.

But there are limits to human endurance. She says, "The first year was pretty difficult. I was exhausted...I knew I was becoming crabby and snappy."

Sandra knew she needed help. She started looking for a home health agency.

Jerry was named in Joe's power of attorney document, and he kept track of his dad's finances. Sandra was conscious of her dad's limited resources, and they all knew they would have to conserve his money to pay for his care. She also knew that her dad would not qualify for Medicaid.

As of 2020, "too many assets" to qualify for Medicaid means having over $2,000 in liquid assets and an income of over $2,349 a month; the amounts were similar in 2014. (Medicaid is not to be confused with Medicare, the medical insurance plan for anyone sixty-five and over. Further information can be found in Appendix 1.)

They checked into Joe's veteran's status. Because Joe was not in the service during a war (he was in between World War II and the Korean War), he did not qualify for certain benefits such as "Aid and Attendance," which is a pension for homebound vets.

Sandra was afraid her dad might run out of money, so she settled on a home health agency offering the lowest price. The company did not have a nurse, only a social worker and aides, which ended up causing even more problems for the family.

The social worker asked Sandra on the phone about her dad's schedule. Sandra named three things, at which point the social worker interrupted her. "This is overwhelming. I did not realize your dad needed so much care."

Puzzled, Sandra responded, "He has Parkinson's disease and is eighty-six years old! What do you want me to do?"

The social worker sighed. "Just write it down and send it to me."

Sandra made the list and sent it off to the social worker, feeling as though they were already off on the wrong foot.

The caregivers came in rotation. One of his favorite aides named Amanda was soft-spoken and patient. But more often, the aides seemed frustrated with Joe. Sometimes, Sandra would hear her dad yelling at the caregiver or the caregiver speaking sharply to him. At first, she would wince inwardly but did not interfere.

Joe said he did not like those people. He did not need them. Finally, it came to a point where Sandra had to tell him to stop being so picky about the caregivers, or he might have to live in a nursing home. This resulted in him becoming more tolerant.

The caregivers would come twice a week during the day and spend every night during the week. It was cheaper if the caregiver could get at least four hours of sleep while staying in the room with Joe, but Sandra said, "That never happened."

Ken and Sandra took turns getting up with Dad on weekends.

The caregivers had been giving Joe his medications, but one of the caregivers just could not keep his medications straight.

When Sandra complained, the social worker said the aides were not supposed to give him meds, which was news to Sandra.

Another caregiver was pleasant, but she spent most of her shift on the phone with her boyfriend.

The whole situation was stressful. Sandra would tell the caregivers her expectations for care, they would come one night, and then they would quit. They said Sandra expected too much.

One night, one of the caregivers was with Joe, and they heard a crash. Joe had fallen. The caregiver said Joe stood up when he was sitting in the commode and fell. However, Sandra had her doubts. This caregiver often yelled at her dad. Sandra suspected the caregiver was abusive, but she did not have proof.

Sandra did file an incident report with the company. She had a good relationship with the owner, who told her, "Your dad needs too much care. Look for another organization where the staff is more skilled."

Sandra started a new search.

Year Three

Sandra's niece Maggie and her son were finally able to move out, creating more space, which was needed for Joe's increasing care needs. As they moved into the third year of caregiving, Sandra hired a new caregiving agency.

She also asked the first agency if she could keep Amanda on; the agency agreed. Amanda was only twenty-two, but she rose above the others in her compassion and ability to connect with Joe. She stayed with Joe for three years. Sandra said, "Amanda was the one we kept the longest. She had extreme patience and kindness and was compassionate and gentle with him."

Due to her experience as a paid caregiver, Amanda knew how one's world shrinks, and the small things we could once control loom big in our minds. It is easy to take out one's frustrations on the caregivers we know best.

Joe was no different; he would express frustration at Amanda because she was the most patient. His complaints were "She doesn't tuck me in right," or "She put too much lotion on my skin." Amanda shared she knew it was not really Joe speaking but his illness, an unusual amount of insight for someone so young.

Amanda was one of five excellent caregivers who took care of Joe.

Two caregivers from the second group stand out in Sandra's mind. They were both kind and compassionate and were willing to make the drive, which was a good distance from their homes. In spite of a couple of early incidents where Joe did not get to the toilet on time, they both continued to care for him until the end.

Sandra then went back to the first caregiving company, which had more experienced caregivers by that time. Sandra paid more money to get their help, and they sent two excellent caregivers. Madison in particular took good care of Joe, although he often told her, "I can never remember your name."

One day, Sandra said, "Dad, do you remember my name?" Joe said, "Of course, you're Natalie!" (Natalie is Sandra's oldest daughter.) Sandra raised her eyebrows in alarm. Then Joe laughed and said, "Sandra, I know your name." Sandra and Madison laughed with him at his joke. They were also relieved he was not showing unusual signs of forgetfulness.

For thirty-two hours a week, Sandra was still taking care of her dad alone. When caregivers were there, she spent time planning, sorting pills, and managing Joe's medical needs such as appointments and obtaining needed equipment and supplies. She also cared for her home, spent time with Ken, and made tasty meals. Even with all of the help, Sandra still frequently transferred Joe to and from sitting and lying down positions. Her back was starting to feel strained. She was not as young as she had been back in the days when she worked in the nursing home.

As time went on, Joe lost more of his independence. He would grow more easily frustrated, at times brooding, or snapping at the caretakers.

To add to the tension, Sandra did not always agree with the caretakers. One nurse said to let Joe skip his exercises one or two days in a row, and then he could see how weak he would become. If Joe were not able to get out of bed, he would learn how important it was to exercise. Hesitatingly, they asked an aide to try her method, and indeed, Joe started to get weaker almost right away. But true to what the nurse predicted Joe was more motivated to do his daily exercises.

During this time, Joe was in the hospital several times. The hospital prepared a healthcare directive for Joe in the event he could not make decisions for himself. Joe did not want to be resuscitated if he was near death, thus his status was "Do Not Resuscitate" or "DNR". He also responded to other questions regarding his care, such as tube-feeding, intubation, or other resuscitative measures.

The first time after he was hospitalized, Joe was sent to a nursing home temporarily for rehabilitation. Sandra visited her dad in rehab and noticed the call button was moved away from him. When she asked why, she was told it was because Joe rang the bell every few minutes.

Joe was so miserable in rehab that the doctor sent him home. Joe did not like the nursing care he received in the home. He liked how his oldest daughter took care of him. Joe was dependent on Sandra. So, Joe came home.

How did Sandra feel about this change in roles? She said, "I wasn't sure why he liked the way I took care of him. I felt like I came across like a drill sergeant. I am afraid I was demeaning. It took a toll on our relationship."

I asked Sandra if her dad ever resented her having to do things for him. Sandra said, "I cannot deny that is the case. I remember the time Dad hurt my feelings in a major way, speaking sharply to me when he could not reach his walker. He was quiet the rest of breakfast, then he said, 'Sandra come here.' He opened his arms wide and said, 'I know you're doing these things to help me. I'm sorry for the way I talked to you,' as he gave me a hug."

Sandra has plenty of good memories of taking care of her dad. Her natural sense of humor would lighten up the day.

Once, Joe told her, "I know you love me Sandra by how well you take care of me."

Sandra said Ken was much more patient. She felt like she had to be the "bad parent" and Ken (and others) were the "good parent." Ken had a way of encouraging Joe to do his exercises with a little prodding, and he would walk with Joe while singing songs like "Amazing Grace." At other times, Ken would just sit with Joe and read to him.

Sandra admits that she was jealous of other family members when they would come over and spend time with Joe. They would play games, look at old pictures, or read to Joe. She felt as though she was focused on the quantity of his life, ensuring he lived longer, while others were focused on the quality of his life.

Even though caregivers came in, Sandra still bore most of the burden. At times, when her husband could see Sandra reaching a breaking point, he would say, "I'm going to take care of Dad Friday night, and you go to a hotel." Ken was her biggest cheerleader.

Hospital Care

One of Joe's most serious falls happened later in the care process when Joe fell, and Sandra could not get him up. She called 911, and Joe spent several days in the hospital.

This time, he hallucinated, which can happen in the later stages of Parkinson's disease. Joe was screaming, "Help me! Help me!" He thought he was all alone, and no one would help him.

Sandra remembers the time the hospital told her the doctor would be in at 10:00 a.m. for a consultation. When Sandra arrived at the hospital a little before 10:00, the nurse told her the doctor had already been to see her dad. "Why couldn't they reach me?" Sandra grimaced in frustration at the memory.

Sandra said, "Trying to plan your visits to see a loved one in the hospital around the doctor's rounds is just frustrating. The doctors are busy, making rounds to many patients, and often dealing with crises. I realized when I missed the doctors, the nurses could fill me in and pass messages on to the physician."

Another time, Joe was in the hospital with several problems, including a neck injury. Sandra was concerned about the way the aide was turning him, so she advised, "You need to support his neck when you move him. If you do it like that, you'll hurt his neck." The aide was offended, and suggested Sandra leave the room. Sandra said, "No, this is my dad, and I want to stay." The nurse was in the room, and he intervened and said Sandra could stay.

Another time, the same aide brought Joe thickened water because he was having difficulty swallowing. The water had ice cubes in it, which is not how thickened water should be served. Sandra let the aide know the ice cubes would melt, and the water would not be thick. Sandra later realized she may have been harsh with the aide, so she went and apologized.

Sandra knew from experience that hospital or nursing home care is difficult for the family, not to mention the nursing staff. As family members, sometimes we need to advocate. At other times, we need to be quiet and apologize freely.

When Joe was in the hospital, it was suggested that he go to a day program for the elderly. Joe was initially opposed to going. The family insisted, and he grew to enjoy the day camp for Parkinson's patients twice a week. He was able to take a mobility bus, so it was a break for Sandra when she could catch up on chores.

Palliative Care

Ken knew Sandra needed more help; she was getting burned out.

Would Joe have to go into a nursing home after all? Did they come this far to relinquish his care now? Was Joe going to run out of money?

Sandra and Ken simply could not supply any more of his care, and although they had caregivers coming in, Joe was getting more medically fragile. Palliative nursing care was suggested, so they signed Joe up for this new level of support.

> Palliative care is specialized care for people living with a serious illness. This type of medical care is focused on improving the quality of life for the patient by finding ways to relieve symptoms. It can also help relieve stress for both the patient and family.

The palliative care nurse held a family meeting with all of the siblings. It was a helpful time where everyone could speak up and share what was on their minds. It also helped them all understand how their dad's disease was progressing and what was needed at this point.

The palliative care nurse came once a week and more often as needed. She would take Joe's vitals and give Sandra medical advice and emotional support.

The palliative care nurse told Sandra, "Your dad has you wrapped around his little finger. He says, 'go,' and you go. 'Jump' and you jump." Sandra now laughs about this, saying, "Well, he was my dad!"

An aide would come and get Joe ready for bed and spend the night. When the aide left in the morning, they gave Sandra the monitor in case Joe had to get up. Another caregiver would come to get Joe up and ready for the day.

One of the advantages of palliative care was that Sandra

could cut down on the drives to her dad's medical appointments. The palliative care nurse would communicate with the doctor, and doctor's visits became much more infrequent. The palliative nurse also helped to get a mobility service lined up for Joe to cut down on driving.

Ken had been giving Joe his baths, but now, the aides took care of the bathing.

One of the effects of Parkinson's disease is the effect on swallowing. Swallow tests showed Joe's swallowing was getting worse, and they diagnosed him with dysphagia.

> "Dysphagia" means swallowing difficulties. Some people with dysphagia have difficulty swallowing certain foods or liquids, and others cannot swallow at all. Signs of dysphagia include coughing or choking when eating or drinking or bringing food back up through the mouth or nose.

To assist with the dysphagia, exercises were prescribed, like singing before he ate. Sandra had him sing "Amazing Grace" with her because it had a good range and Joe knew the words. Some of the aides did not want to sing, so Sandra taped her dad and herself singing "Amazing Grace" for times she was not home. The aide played it for him, and Joe sang along.

Now when Sandra hears "Amazing Grace," she gets a lump in her throat, thinking of the times she and her dad sang together.

Joe was put on a pureed food diet, which he liked, even though it meant he could not have cookies. He had been receiving meals from the Community Assistance Emergency Program (CEAP), but since they did not supply pureed food, Sandra found another company to deliver pureed food.

I asked Sandra if it was hard to see her dad get weaker and more dependent. She replied with a catch in her voice, "Yes, it was emotionally difficult to see Dad go downhill."

I asked, "Sandra, what did you find the most difficult?"

Sandra said, "I had the most difficulty when I did not feel supported or if people were criticizing me. Those old tapes from childhood played in my mind." Sandra continued, "Those were just moments of discouragement in time that passed quickly. I did not feel like giving up, but at times, I was beside myself."

Hospice

Several months went by, and while the palliative care services were helpful, they were still not enough. The palliative nurse advocated for Joe to go to hospice because hospice provides more nursing care and extra services. Joe did not want to go to hospice because he thought it meant he would die. They had to explain to Joe it did not mean he would die; it would be an advantage to all of the family.

> Hospice care is designed to support people in the final phase of life. It focuses on comfort and quality of life rather than on finding a cure. The goal is for patients to be comfortable and free of pain so they can enjoy the rest of their life.

Sandra found out later the main reason the palliative nurse wanted Joe to start receiving hospice care was because she was worried about Sandra who was showing signs of exhaustion.

Hospice offered Joe a number of services:

- A music therapist came in often and played for Joe, which he enjoyed.
- Joe refused to get a massage when the therapist came in, so they gave Sandra the massage!
- Twice a volunteer came in to read to Joe. However, Sandra had more free time to spend with her dad, so she took over the quiet reading times with him.
- Physical therapy came on a regular basis.
- An aide came in to give him a bath at least twice a week.

The hospice care team recommended they send Joe to respite care once in a while to give Sandra and Ken a short break. This could either be in a home that provided respite care or a nursing home. They tried respite care on three different occasions.

The first place Joe went to could not figure out the difference between his compression socks and regular socks, so they just used regular socks. As a result, Joe could not walk while he was there, and he came home much weaker. Sandra admits this home may have been the cheapest place she looked into.

The second time they tried respite care was in a nursing home. In spite of it being a reputable place, after a week, Joe came home with a bedsore that never completely went away.

They tried one more place. Sandra and the hospice team liked it, but Joe did not. He reported there was a lady there who was loud and talked a lot.

Sandra knew in her heart no one would take care of her dad quite like her. This knowledge kept her going.

Joe was on hospice care for a year, which is unusual because it is generally meant for people with six months or less to live. The family and medical team were considering taking him off hospice the day disaster hit.

Time and Again

Madison, the aide whose name Joe could never remember, quit about three weeks before Joe had his final fall. She said she was uncomfortable taking care of him as he was getting weaker and needed two people to move him.

Sandra talked to a third caregiving company, which came out and evaluated Joe. That day, Joe was having an exceptionally good day. The social worker, nurse, and administrator all said Joe did not need two people to move him. They offered to send an orderly who could lift him alone. However, that was much more expensive.

One of the regular caregivers was at the house on a Friday caring for Joe. He went to sit in his chair while the caregiver stood on the side to help him. Suddenly, Joe pitched forward and fell on the floor. The caregiver was unable to catch him. Sandra heard the cry and ran into the living room. There she found her dad bleeding on the floor, and the caregiver standing over him. Sandra told the caregiver to call 911 while she grabbed a towel to try to stop the bleeding. Time stood still for her.

When the paramedics came, the caregiver cried, certain it was her fault. The ambulance whisked Joe off to the hospital emergency room where Sandra met him. Sandra was white and shaky. One of the nurses asked if she needed to sit down, but Sandra said she was okay. There was a long wait in the emergency room while they found Joe had cracked a bone in his neck.

Sandra stayed in the hospital with him for several nights, and other family members came to visit.

Joe would eat a few bites of softened food at a time, and one sibling wondered why they were not giving him fluids intravenously. But according to Joe's healthcare directive, Joe did not want artificial support. He was nearly ninety years old and had suffered from Parkinson's disease for over seven years.

Thoughts flew through Sandra's mind:

Would they send Dad home with a neck brace? Would they lose all of his caregivers because they may not be able to take care of him? Would she have to do all of the caretaking herself? Could she even do so?

Her dad asked, "Am I still welcome at your house, Sandra?"

"Yes, Dad, of course, you are welcome."

This was Joe's way of asking if he was going to live and be able to go home. In her heart, Sandra just did not know if that would happen. Her dad wanted to keep fighting, but he was getting weaker.

The medical team said the fracture in his neck could heal, but he was unable to eat much. Sandra was able to get him to eat small, pureed meals.

Family came into the hospital more frequently. They read to Joe, sang to him, held his hand, and told their dad and grandpa how much they loved him.

The caregiver who had been there when Joe fell felt guilty about the fall. She asked if she could visit Joe. Sandra left the room when the caregiver came so that she could have a private conversation with Joe as she asked for his forgiveness.

Sandra also felt guilty. Should she have had two caregivers? Or have an orderly come around the clock? Could she have done something to prevent the fall?

On Saturday, Sandra had a good day with her dad. She said it was a gift from the Lord that she did not have to be the caregiver, the drill sergeant. She could just be his daughter again. Joe was more alert, and she read to him from an archaeological book he loved and the Bible.

Joe was a minster and life-long child of God, but he still expressed fear of dying, as our human nature fears the unknown.

On Sunday, Sandra gave her dad two bites of thickened water, and then he fell asleep. After a while, Sandra went into the public bathroom where she sobbed. She realized he was only eating to appease her. The stress, the scare of the fall, and the realization that her dad was likely in his last days hit her all at once.

Sandra called everyone in the family and told them it was time to come and see their dad and grandpa. Sunday night, his four children came, and nearly all of the grandchildren. By this time, Joe was a grandfather, great-grandfather, and great-great-grandfather!

Joe slept most of the day. Sandra asked if he would wake up, and the nurse said probably not. However, when one of the daughters held his hand and said, "I love you, Dad," he woke up and smiled at her. She holds this special moment in her heart.

Joe fidgeted in his sleep, and the nurses said it was because he was in pain. They gave him morphine to help lessen the pain. Hospice continued to come in while Joe was in the hospital to play music and offer a massage to Sandra.

The next day, Joe was more alert. Sandra had a good day with him, as did some of the other family members who came to visit.

The physician's assistant came in and said Joe would not be going home as he likely had aspiration pneumonia. They took off Joe's neck brace, treated his bedsore, and administered morphine. Comfort was most important.

Joe went to sleep that night, and afterward, he only woke up to get pain medication. Time passed slowly as Sandra and her siblings sat quietly by Joe's side.

Wednesday, Joe slipped into the arms of Jesus, where there is no more fear, no more suffering, and no more death.

"Precious in the sight of the Lord is the death of his faithful servants." – Psalm 116:15

Advice

Sandra, would you take your dad in again?

Totally. Dad enriched our lives and made us better.

Was there ever a time you wished you had not taken care of your dad?

No, never.

What advice would you give someone who was thinking about taking a relative into their home?

For someone to do this, they have to be motivated by love. You have to know your own limitations, and you have to know what the deal-breaker would be for you.

What would have been your "deal-breaker" that would have ended the home care for your dad?

If we could have no longer kept him safe. For example, if he wandered outside or insisted on walking without his walker. Also, if Ken or I had had a major health change, we may not have been able to care for him. Although, we were fortunate, and we both remained healthy.

Any other advice?

People need to know they will need help. Learn what is available and what you can afford. If your loved one gets sicker, know how you will provide care for them.

What was the most important key to your successful caregiving for your dad?

Knowing my husband supported me and willingly helped. I also knew other family members were there for Dad, and they encouraged me.

Author Reflections

Sandra and Ken have a strong faith, and they often say that by the grace of God, they were able to serve their beloved dad in his final years.

Would you like to evaluate a potential home care situation for a loved one in your life? See Appendix 2, "Caregiving Checklist for Home Care" to help in the decision-making process.

Chapter 4
Friendship

"Time and good friends are two things that become more valuable the older you get."
– https://livelifehappy.com

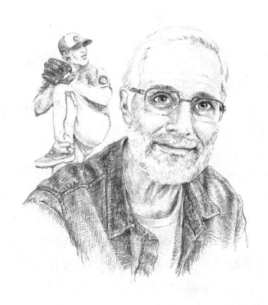

Introduction

According to AARP®, there were sixteen million family caregivers in 2017, and 40 percent were male.[2] The numbers do not include men who help care for friends or non-family members. And of course, numbers do not touch on the joys and heartache of caretaking.

I wondered, do men have a unique perspective? Are they more or less caring than women? Of course, one story does not apply to all men just as one story of a female caregiver does not apply to all women. However, there are lessons we can learn from Phil's point of view, and the tale of two men who were as close or closer than brothers.

Speed and Agility

Phil and Wally enjoyed one of those rare friendships spanning decades. They met when their families were young. Their wives and children also became friends, and they shared many good times while their families grew, and their children spread their wings.

Phil and his wife Linda were there when Wally's first wife tragically died of cancer, and he was left with two young children. And they celebrated with him when he met his second wife Kathleen, a widow with two children.

Snowmobiling was Phil and Wally's favorite activity, a great way to enjoy northern winters. Sometimes, they would find nearby trails for an afternoon outing. Often, they went on a "guys" weekend with Wally's brothers to their family cabin further north. There the snow fell in abundance, and the air was crisp and cold. Through smooth trails and rough woods, they explored the great outdoors.

Sometimes, especially on the Martin Luther King Jr. long weekend, the families would head to a resort. Here, the snowmobilers could take to the trails, come in for a hot meal, and head out again. The non-snowmobilers enjoyed a warm fire, talks, and games. The family bonds grew strong during these memorable days.

Snowmobiling requires strength and flexibility to maneuver on the trails. It also requires good visual acuity and alertness to avoid dangerous situations. The driver must be agile enough to keep control of the vehicle to avoid getting injured or hurting others. It is a challenge they relished.

Much later, Phil and Wally looked back at those adventures with longing and nostalgia because there came a day when Wally could no longer manage his day-to-day activities, much less control his beloved "sled." Fortunately, Wally had a friend by his side through a whole new set of challenges.

Phil was used to loss, as much as any of us can adapt to losing loved ones on this earth. He had lost three close friends and he was a caretaker for his dad, who died in his mid-sixties. After that, he aided his mother, initially in regard to finances. Later, his mom developed dementia and cancer, and Phil became the primary caregiver for her. He also had an uncle who died in his mid-forties. Phil was no stranger to grief.

Phil worked in the medical field, giving him an advantage in understanding the physical effects of illness. His unique outlook affected him in a distinct way, combining knowledge of how a person may feel, how the disease could progress, and empathy as both a professional and personal caregiver.

Wally was a savvy businessman and a persuasive negotiator. As a collector, he found good deals everywhere. He and his wife

Kathleen loved to travel, almost as much as they loved family gatherings. When he was not snowmobiling in the winter, he was fly-fishing in the summer, another activity requiring agility and attention.

Wally and Phil supported each other through life's ups and downs. For example, Phil's mom lived in a small town in southern Minnesota. When it became apparent his mom could no longer care for herself, Wally helped Phil locate a place close to their house, where his mom was able to spend the rest of her life.

When Wally was in his fifties, he started noticing symptoms such as tremors, limb stiffness, impaired balance, and slower movement. At first, he tried to ignore the warning signs; maybe he was only tired or aging. After a while, his family started to make comments. He could not hide his symptoms from Kathleen, who was a nurse and knew her husband well.

When the diagnosis of Parkinson's disease was confirmed, they were both relieved and apprehensive. Relieved because it explained Wally's symptoms. Also, it was not imminently fatal; people often live for years with Parkinson's. Apprehensive because they knew about the disease and how it might progress. In the beginning, Wally could still do his normal activities of working, spending time with his family, fishing, and snowmobiling—of course. However, as time went on, many activities became more difficult.

One of the stranger side effects for Wally was an increased need to shop all of the time. He would come home with unusual purchases, much to Kathleen's surprise. She would call Phil, who could pick up the extra items and return them to Costco. Wally did not seem to notice his new items were missing.

Activities requiring motor skills and attention became more difficult. Not only do these changes present challenges and frequent adjustments, but Parkinson's patients can also become a danger to others. Wally concluded that he needed to stop driving as the medications made him tired. When they went on trips to the cabin, Phil drove while Wally slept.

Wally had served in the National Guard. He did a lot of hunting in his earlier years and owned a number of firearms. Phil recounted one time later on in Wally's disease progression when Wally's disability could have been dangerous.

Phil, Wally, and Wally's brothers were at the cabin for a late summer outing. The brothers were hunters. Wally enjoyed patiently waiting in the woods for a big buck, and he was nearly always a sure shot.

The brothers grabbed their firearms, heading to a gravel pit to shoot.

Phil stated, "I was never in the military, and firearms were not a part of my life. I had shot them a few times when I was young, but for the most part, guns were foreign to me. On that trip, when Wally took up his handgun, he was having significant tremors. I was uncomfortable, thinking about what could happen if Wally were not thinking clearly and had a firearm available."

Wally's son must have had the same thoughts because he removed the firearms from the house.

"Be cautious with firearms and other weapons in the house of someone who is not capable of handling them anymore," Phil advised. "The impact of what they can do can be so dangerous. This is one thing I strongly advise."

As the years progressed, the changes became more pronounced, and after a while, the effect of Parkinson's forced Wally to leave much of what he enjoyed behind. His inability to snowmobile was especially difficult. At this point, it became necessary to prescribe antidepressants.

The Relief Pitcher

Wally and Kathleen's home had two floors with all of the bedrooms upstairs. Wally went from slowing down on the stairs, to holding the railing to go one step at a time, to avoiding the stairs as often as possible. Tearfully, Kathleen asked Wally's brothers and Phil to help remodel their house so that Wally could stay at home. Moving Wally to another living situation at this young age was unthinkable.

The alterations required research and creative problem-solving. Some could be done in a weekend, but other changes needed to be hired out to professionals. The living room was turned into a bedroom, and the bathroom was redone to accommodate his needs. Handles and grab bars were placed around the walls, and they bought a lift chair.

Kathleen was a nurse and was determined to care for her husband. However, like many caregivers, she had trouble remembering to care for herself.

Phil said, "Wally's disease really got to Kathleen. She got into it much too deeply than was good for her mental health. She was sliding and had her own medical issues.

"I would call her and tell her she needed to get out, recharge her batteries. At first, this was difficult. She did not want to impose on others. It was difficult to convince her to leave and find something enjoyable with her friends.

"What Kathleen needed was a relief pitcher, and I was that person. As a caregiver, you cannot just suffer in silence. It will kill you."

Phil told Kathleen she could call him any time to come over so she could have a break. She began to take him up on the offer.

When Phil stopped over, the guys would enjoy a ball game, reminisce about snowmobiling trips and mishaps, or talk about the latest accounts of their now-grown children. Kathleen often left lunch or snacks handy.

Phil recounts when Wally started hallucinating, which happens to approximately thirty percent of Parkinson's patients. He started seeing bugs coming out of the toilet to get him. He reported seeing people both inside and outside of the house. Phil said, "When he would drag me to the window to show me 'the people,' my first impulse was to argue with him. But I learned quickly not to argue because that is what he was seeing."

While the "people" were just shadows, they can seem real to a person whose brain is playing tricks on their eyes.

While Wally could still get into a car, the two guys would go out to their favorite restaurant for lunch. Wally was having trouble eating and swallowing. Sometimes, food got stuck in his throat or excess saliva would cause drooling. Phil recalled, "I had to work hard not to feel uncomfortable for him with the other patrons around. You just have to look past appearances. If people are judgmental, so be it. It is what it is."

Transition

Parkinson's continued to creep throughout Wally's nervous system, and he became progressively worse. Wally worried about his wife, who had already lost one spouse. His children had lost their mom to cancer at a young age. How would they handle if he did not make it to an old age as he always thought? Wally desperately wished he did not have the disease, and he hoped not to deteriorate any faster. But wishes do not halt the course of disease, and an unsettled acceptance seemed the only way to manage the inevitable. Anti-depressants also helped him cope.

When Wally needed to use a wheelchair nearly all of the time, he and Kathleen had to admit she could no longer care for him at home. Even with her nursing experience, lifting or transferring him became dangerous to both of them. They needed a place where he could get more constant care. Phil and Linda helped Kathleen find a place for Wally where he could get help with daily activities and his medical needs.

Together, they moved Wally into an assisted living and memory care facility close to Kathleen's house. There they offered mind-engaging activities, exercises, art, gardening, and delicious food. Nursing care was on-sight. While Kathleen struggled with guilt, she could at least be at peace knowing Wally was well taken care of.

With Wally in the facility, Phil no longer had to convince Kathleen to let him help. He was able to visit Wally as his time permitted. Cognitively, Wally knew people and maintained his ability to have conversations. His symptoms were more physical: shaking, rigidity, and paralysis primarily on the right (fortunately, Wally was left-handed.) Wally's main problem was he had trouble with his brain telling his muscles to move.

Wally was always happy to see Phil, and the staff also enjoyed his visits. When the weather was agreeable, Wally and Phil went out to the courtyard where Wally would try to walk. After a while, this too became more and more difficult due to the limitations of Parkinson's. Wally fell a couple of times when Phil was there visiting. It was difficult to witness this former National Guard soldier, hunter, fisherman and snowmobiler not able to walk or even stand. After a while, Wally used the wheelchair all of the time.

Eventually, Wally had to move to a nursing home where he could receive full-time care. Although he suffered from depression at the end, he fought the monster for nineteen years. Phil smiled at the memories. "I give him a lot of credit for not letting the disease define him. Wally was a great example of how a person dealt with something so debilitating. He did not crawl in a hole; he fought it."

Although Phil was used to caretaking with family members, witnessing the decline of such a good friend his age gave him a new perspective, and it was unnerving.

At age seventy, Wally succumbed to the devastation Parkinson's wrought on his body and mind. He was a true soldier to the end. Wally's obituary read, "Wally courageously battled Parkinson's disease for nearly twenty years. With Kathleen by his side, he continued to enjoy life. Kathleen's unrelenting love and devotion have been unmatched."

And fortunately, Kathleen had Phil as a relief pitcher for the times she was weary, broken, or just needed a break.

Advice

Phil, were you able to help the family with any other challenges?

Wally always took care of the outdoors; he loved the lawn and his riding lawn mower. When he could no longer balance or maneuver the machine, he would still change the oil. At times, I helped with the lawn. After Wally died, I spent time teaching Kathleen how to operate the John Deere mower.

Kathleen and Wally handled their own finances. I would have helped had they asked, but that was their private family business. Wally was financially savvy. Kathleen had worked most of her life and knew she would need to protect her resources. She hired an elder care financial advisor and an attorney.

The laws are complicated. Get professional advice to protect the surviving spouse. When you look at the cost of living in a care facility, it is astronomical and getting worse. The survivor has to cover their needs as well.

What else would you advise caregivers?

A lot of it depends on the relationship with the person. I had a long relationship with Wally. While it was sad to see his situation, I was able to overlook a lot of the side effects of the disease and see the person.

This is one thing I advise people: you have to look past the bad. I am just stubborn enough to say, "It is what it is," and you just have to accept the situation.

Depression is a big problem for people with these diseases. You are losing the ability to take care of yourself, and it is a hard pill to swallow. That is where a neurologist comes in. They have to be the ones to make the call on how to treat the mental health issues.

The patient's medical team may also need to make that sort of call for the caregivers. If the primary caregiver is showing signs of depression, they may need the help of medication in order to cope and not go batty. At a minimum, the patient's medical professional should be ready to refer the primary caregiver to resources or their own primary doctor.

Do you see any differences in how you as a man experience caregiving versus how you see women doing so? How do you think caregiving is different from a man's point of view?

I do not want to sound sexist. Women are more into caregiving. Often, they choose it as an occupation. From a male point of view, men have to make more of an effort to be this kind of a caregiver. Men are supposed to be independent, self-reliant. You have to deliberately see a situation where people are needy, and men tend to shy away from the situation.

You just do it. Everybody deals mentally with this type of situation differently. Some people just do not want to help. To try and change people and say, 'Step up to the plate'— maybe yes and maybe no. In some instances, guys just will not take on that type of caregiving.

Did your faith play a role in your caregiving?

A line out of a sermon by a priest named Ralph has stuck with me. Ralph told how his mother told him, "Ralph, pray for a happy death." It seems counterintuitive; death is not a happy experience in people's minds, but a happy death, it is what I hope for.

When people do not have a sense there is something better than existence here on earth, they have a tough time. You have to have a spot to land. We have to believe in God's unlimited love for us. In return, we are asked to return God's love to our fellow man in their hour of need.

In retrospect, how do you view your role as Wally's caregiver?

In a sense, maybe I filled in a vacuum that was there. I look at it as incumbent upon myself to help others because someday, I will need help. You have to live your life as a good example for your kids and others. You have to walk the walk, do the right thing, and be there if somebody needs help. It may cost you a little bit in time and effort, but there for the grace of God go I.

I felt like it was my duty to help out as much as I could. We were friends for over forty years. Caring for Wally when he needed help gave me a sense of purpose.

We should not let people suffer needlessly because they do not have the help. You have to look out for each other.

Phil reflected a bit more on Wally's situation, and his voice caught in his throat. It was an emotional display I had not expected, but neither did it surprise me.

Author Reflections

I have known Phil and his family for years; however I developed a deeper respect for the character of this man as I learned how he faithfully cared for his friend. We should all be so fortunate.

People are individuals, both men and women have served as outstanding caregivers; both men and women have rejected the caregiving role. It is important to support and respect any person who offers a hand of friendship to the care receiver.

Chapter 5

Paradise Lost and Paradise Found

"To care for those who once cared for us is one of the highest honors."
– Tia Walker, *The Inspired Caregiver: Finding Joy While Caring for Those You Love*

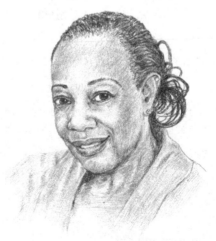

Introduction

This book was written in 2020, a year of turmoil, not only with the pandemic but also with racial tension. I wanted to include a story about healthcare in ethnic minority populations.

I was led to Jean by her daughter. Jean is an incredible woman who does not let anything deter her from taking care of her own. I found an overcomer, and I learned what she believes was the root cause of healthcare disparity in her family.

Growing Up in Gary

She had the dream plan, and it was about to come true. Jean, an attractive middle-aged single parent, was about to see her three children launched into early adulthood. It was time for her next life phase, and it was a great plan!

After attending a year of college, her son decided he preferred full-time work and was living on his own. Her two daughters were only fourteen months apart in age. When her oldest daughter was accepted into Hawaii Pacific University, the girls were in a quandary because they could not live without each other. The youngest daughter, smart and ambitious, knew she was ready to graduate from high school a year early, and she was also accepted into Hawaii Pacific University. Ecstatic, the girls packed their suitcases and together headed off to their college adventure.

Normally, Jean, like any parent, would have been sad to see her kids head out, but they had hatched a plan. She emptied her apartment and moved in with a girlfriend temporarily. Within six months, Jean would follow her daughters to the warm, sunny utopia. After living through the Indiana and Minnesota winters, Hawaii was to be her paradise.

Until the dream shattered around her like pieces of broken glass.

What led Jean to her broken dreams?

Let us back up and visit Gary, Indiana, where Jean's family moved.

Gary was formed in 1906 by the U.S. Steel Corporation where they built Gary Works, a massive steel plant. Gary attracted a diverse population, including African Americans from the Great Migration, where over six million black people moved to northern cities to obtain employment. Anyone with nothing more than a sixth-grade education could work in the steel mills, making a good living.

Harold and Grace worked their way to Gary as part of the Great Migration. Harold worked in the steel mills. He was a hard worker and relished the time home with his wife and their only child, Victoria. Grace, a beautiful and gracious woman, kept the home, and made many friends in Gary. She always wore a dress or matching ensemble when leaving home, and in turn Grace dressed Victoria like Shirley Temple in frilly dresses and patent leather baby doll shoes. When she grew up, Victoria continued to "dress to the nines." (To the nines is an idiom meaning "perfection" or "to the highest degree.") Grace made certain the females in the family knew her motto: "Women should never leave home without their hair done-up and being dressed nicely."

Grace and Harold adored Victoria; they wanted their only daughter to seek higher education. But Victoria was growing up fast, and much to her parent's distress, she met the man of her dreams when she was only eighteen, a senior in high school. He had been drafted and was leaving for the Navy, so they married and moved to California where he was stationed. She quickly became pregnant, and he went out to sea. Once he returned to California, they had their second child and then the third child, each two years apart.

They moved back home to Gary when he was discharged from the service. There, Jean was born, four years after child number three.

Too often, war-time veterans found civilian life difficult, and many World War II veterans had what they called "shell-shock." Now, we know it as post-traumatic stress disorder. Victoria and her husband had their own set of problems, and their marriage turned rocky. They already had four children, and while they teetered on divorce, two more were born. They eventually parted ways.

Victoria was left to raise her six children alone. Without a father in the home, the family lived in poverty. Victoria required her children to go to church and do well in school. Religion and education were not optional.

As was typical for that generation, there was never a discussion of the "birds and the bees" (sex education). Jean said, "I was not offered guidelines for choosing a man to be your husband based on how he treated a woman. Instead, the focus was on what he had to offer financially."

Jean's mother had rules for her home that were to be followed regardless of the age of her children. Curfew was at 10:00

p.m. unless you were at work. Out of respect for her mom's rules and her determination to be independent, Jean moved out on her own at age eighteen. With limited guidance on how to navigate life, Jean became a single mom at nineteen years of age. The relationship with her son's father ended shortly after her son was born. Jean was determined to be a better single mother than her mother was—whatever that looked like.

Jean met a man a few years later. This time, she was sure he was "Mr. Right," and they romantically discussed getting married. Jean became pregnant and gave birth to a beautiful baby girl. But not all was right because "Mr. Wrong" became alarmingly controlling.

Just as Jean decided she was going to get out of this relationship, she discovered at her annual physical that she was pregnant once again. Jean was devastated. Not only was she looking for a way to get out of this relationship, but her daughter was also only six months old, and her son was three.

Jean had no idea of what she would do with three children as a single parent. As much as she was determined to not be like her mom, history was repeating itself. The unfortunate truth, however, was that Jean still lived in Gary, Indiana, and Gary was not the worker's dream it had been.

> Richard Hatcher, the first black mayor of Gary, had been elected on November 7th, 1967. He served until 1987 and was a vocal civil rights advocate. He fought racism and corruption and experienced a fair amount of controversy.

In the 1970s, with Jean as a young mother of three, the U.S. was plunged into a recession, and the steel industry collapsed like a house of cards as more steel production went overseas.

Mayor Hatcher continued to fight, but Gary spun into an economic spiral, putting many people out of work. In the early 1970s, Gary Works employed over thirty-thousand people, but by the end of the 1980s, only six thousand remained. The economy was devasted, and poverty ran rampant. Many of the white businesses moved out of Gary to nearby Merrillville, Indiana.[3]

Jean and her family were not immune to the economic and societal problems of Gary. She lived in public housing because it was affordable, and Jean worked for the Postal Service for a short time. She was determined to care for her family. However, with jobs being scarce and healthcare poor, Jean knew she needed to find a way out for her children.

I asked Jean about discrimination in Gary. She stated, "As far as discrimination, it was present, but it wasn't going to deter me from what I was going to do. Healthcare was a problem, not just because we were black but because we were poor. I went to a neighboring predominantly white city for healthcare and received good treatment."

Jean went on to report, "Gary was bad because the economy was bad. There were also people moving to Gary from other places. Many of them did not have the same values and love of Gary many of us who were born and raised there had. It no longer had anything to offer, and I knew I would have to look elsewhere to successfully support and raise my three young children, ages two, three, and six."

Jean knew a family who lived in Minneapolis, Minnesota, where the economy was better, and more jobs were available. They offered to help her if she ever decided to relocate. On June 16th, 1980, Jean called her mom and her siblings to let them know she was moving to Minnesota.

Jean knew the father of her two daughters would never agree to her relocating with the children, so she planned a fast getaway, packing their suitcases and gritting her teeth. Her family came to the bus station to say their good-byes, and Jean and the three wide-eyed children headed off to Minnesota.

Minnesota

At first, they stayed with friends. Jean states, "I found a job right away, and have had work ever since I moved here. I had my own apartment by August of that year."

Jean raised her three children in the Minneapolis suburbs. For ten years she was a city bus driver. Then one day, she reported to work and took a fall in oil splattered on the floor by her bus. This caused an injury, which ended her driving career. She would have to find a new job.

Next, she went to work in an office at a school but took a significant pay cut. Somehow, they got by, but it was a daily struggle for Jean. Poverty hovered at their door.

Before she knew it, her kids were about to graduate from high school, and Jean faced the possibility of being alone.

Her one regret was leaving her mom back in Gary. The healthcare was dreadful, and the crime rate was out of control. Jean and her mom talked often. Jean tried to talk her mom into moving to Minnesota.

Victoria insisted, "Gary is my home. I'm not leaving!"

The day everything changed was the day Jean received a call from her mom who reported she was going to have brain surgery for a tumor.

"Mom, are you sure? When did they discover you have a brain tumor?" Jean had a lot of questions, and the answers were slow to come.

Finally, she got the true story out of Victoria. "I've been having headaches for a while. The doctor figures it is a brain tumor."

What? Did Victoria have any type of scan? Jean discovered, no, a scan had not been performed. Healthcare was still bleak in Gary, and tests such as a computed tomography (CAT) scan were considered a luxury. The doctor was merely going off the fact she had headaches.

Jean drove to Gary and brought her mother to the University of Minnesota (U of MN) hospital for a complete physical. She would need a CAT scan to determine the cause of the headaches. Victoria was claustrophobic, so when she went for the scan, the kind doctor accompanied her and held her hand.

Jean said, "It was God watching over her. I knew Mom had good treatment. The doctor knew she was claustrophobic and took care of her." She knew her mom was in the right place.

It was there they discovered that her headaches were stress-related and not from a tumor. They all breathed a huge sigh of relief.

The good part of this experience was Jean finally convinced her mother to move to Minnesota.

Victoria was outgoing and loved life. Relocating to Minnesota was the best thing she could have ever done. Here, there was good clean, safe living. As Victoria did not drive, public transportation allowed her to come and go as she pleased, not having to wait on anyone to take her places. She was hired as a receptionist at a hospital where everyone loved her smile and friendly nature. She loved to travel and took every opportunity to visit new places. A true people person, Victoria cared about her community and knew all of the neighbors. Believing in giving back, she served as an election judge every year.

With her daughters in Hawaii, Jean was living with a friend trying to save money to relocate to Hawaii in December. She received an opportunity of a lifetime to work for the Federal Court. Jean took the job with the intent of keeping it a few months and possibly transferring to the court in Hawaii.

Life Change

Three weeks into the job, Jean's supervisor came to her desk. "Someone is out front to see you." Jean was surprised as visitors did not frequently come to the courthouse. Out front was her youngest brother who had just gotten out of the military and relocated to Minnesota to be with Jean and the kids.

"Mom had an accident; you need to come now."

Jean left her job, and they rushed to the hospital where she found her mom in bad shape. Crossing a familiar busy street, Victoria had been hit by a school bus. They later found out the driver attempted to race through the crosswalk ahead of Victoria and hit her hard. Even now, Jean becomes sick to her stomach whenever she thinks of her precious mom being helplessly slammed into by the big bus.

Victoria had six brain contusions, a ruptured spleen, and six broken ribs. She was in so much pain she wanted to die. They did emergency surgery to remove the spleen, but there was nothing to be done for the broken ribs or the contusions. Healing would be a matter of time.

Fortunately, Victoria was at a city hospital near Jean's work. Jean would go check on her mom before work, during lunch, and after work. The friend she was staying with lived outside of the city, so late in the evening, Jean would catch the bus home to her friend's house.

Forty-eight hours after the surgery, Victoria moved to a non-intensive care hospital room. Jean had gone home to clean up. Upon her return to the hospital, she found her mom slurring her words. Did she have a stroke? Jean bustled off to find the nurse. It turned out they had given Victoria medications for epilepsy to help her brain contusions. She had been given too high a dose and was overdosing on the potent medication.

Jean's heart sank, and anxiety and guilt plagued her mind. Why hadn't she been there? How could she be two places at once? What to do? What if they gave her mom something else toxic?

Such thoughts can go around and around in the caregiver's mind. It is easy to feel responsible for everything that happens to a loved one.

Jean realized she would need to get more actively involved in her mom's care, even while she was in the hospital.

Cleanliness was important to Victoria, and she passed this onto her family. When Jean arrived on day four, she noticed her mom's gown was dirty with dried food. Jean helped her change, and from then on, Jean knew she would have to get her mom out of that hospital. In addition, Victoria was not getting relief from the pain of the broken ribs, and Jean knew something else had to be done.

Jean contacted their family doctor, who knew both Jean and her mom. Jean explained her mom's situation, asking for help.

The doctor said, "I'm running a marathon Sunday. I cannot practice at that hospital, but I'll stop by for a 'visit' with your mom after the marathon."

True to his word, he stopped by to see Victoria. After the visit, he recommended Jean talk to the attending physician and request she transfer Victoria to the hospital where he had practitioner rights. He could then be in charge of her care.

A week passed, and with Victoria out of immediate danger, some of Victoria's kids wanted to move her to a nursing home for rehabilitation.

Victoria pleaded to Jean, "Please don't put me in a nursing home. I will die there!"

Jean was in a quandary; she wanted to honor her mom, but, as she stated, "I did not want to be the sibling who started a fight." Maybe her attorney could advise her? She asked him if she needed power of attorney to make the decision on where to move her mom.

The attorney advised, "No, you don't need it if the other hospital agrees to take her in. Just go ahead and move her."

The doctor released Victoria from the hospital for rehab. This allowed Jean to have her mom moved by medical transport to the hospital where their family doctor had practitioner rights. She let her siblings know where their mom was after the move.

The new hospital only had a room available in the hospice wing. Jean agreed to the room because she knew her mother was too ill to be concerned about what wing she would be in.

Jean knew she would be the one to take care of her mom and was glad her kids were out of the house. Even though the new hospital was only two miles away from Jean's work, it was through city traffic and was inconvenient for Jean. However, she knew that in this new hospital, her mom would be under the care of the doctor she trusted, so Jean was determined to make it work.

Jean's new workplace did not grant Jean time off to take care of her mom. She had already taken a week off while her mom was first in the hospital, but she needed her job and did not want to risk losing her paycheck and benefits. Jean was tasked with learning a new job along with figuring out how to care for her mom. In the beginning, she would get a ride to the hospital after work, stay until 9:00 or 10:00 p.m., and then get a ride back downtown where she would take the bus home. She would return the next morning, leaving in time to get to work by 8:00 a.m.

> This was prior to the Family Medical Leave Act (FMLA) being made law. The FMLA entitles eligible employees to take unpaid, job-protected leave for certain family and medical reasons without losing their jobs.

Because it was in the hospice wing, the level of care was different than it would have been in a regular hospital room. Hospice is focused on comfort care. One of the nurses had let Jean know that it would be wise to have someone with Victoria at all times as they were short-staffed and would not be able to provide her with the time and attention she would need.

For example, the nurse informed Jean they would only bathe Victoria once a week. Jean knew a weekly bath would never be acceptable to her mom. So, they loaded her into a wheelchair and took her to the wheel-in shower where Jean bathed her mom daily.

Clothes were another issue. All of her mom's clothes were too dressy for the hospital, and the thought of leaving Victoria in hospital gowns was a morale buster. Jean bought her mom sweatpants and slip-on shirts and brought Victoria's own night-gowns for the night. Jean learned all she could about how to care for her mom. Jean monitored her mother's care and served as her mom's personal aide.

During one of Victoria's first evenings in the new hospital, a nurse came in to give her medication. Jean was there and asked, as she did routinely, "What medication are you giving Mom?"

"Insulin," replied the nurse.

Jean's eyes grew large. "Mom is not diabetic!" This incident led to Jean learning what medicines her mother was actually pre-scribed, the dose of each medication, and how often she was to receive it.

From that point on, Jean studied how to use medications; she learned their basic use and became adept at tracking and managing doses.

Jean cleaned the room at the new hospital daily with an antiseptic cleaner and washed the bathroom down. She wanted her mom to feel at home and safe.

But Victoria was suffering, and the pain was unbearable. She prayed God would take her life.

The main order of business was for the doctor to find a way to stop Victoria's pain from the broken ribs. The family doctor soon found a combination of medications that helped control the pain without making Victoria sick from the medicine. This was the turning point for Victoria's recovery.

One sign of hope was when her mom clearly did not want to die anymore. She said, "If I lay in bed all the time, I will die." She sat in the chair as much as possible.

Jean also learned about nutrition for her mom, as many hospice patients do not have much of an appetite, and there is not much of a need to balance their nutrition. Jean came to rely on a protein drink for her mom and kept it well-stocked at the hospital.

Victoria's seventieth birthday was approaching. The family loved celebrations, and this birthday was extra special. Unfortunately, Victoria was still in the hospital, so her siblings and her children all came to town to celebrate with her in the hospital room. All agreed it was a blessing she was not only alive but also mentally and emotionally well considering all she had been through.

With her siblings there with Mom, Jean decided to sneak out to grab a bite to eat. To her surprise, when she came back, all her siblings were gone. Puzzled, Jean sat down next to her mom, waiting for them to return. They came back smiling and laughing.

"We had the best time! The Twins Fest is right down from the hospital on the plaza. We even saw some of the players!"

(Twins Fest is an annual fundraiser for the Minnesota Twins Baseball Team Community Fund.)

Jean said, "I could see how this was going to go!" She smiled when she said this, knowing her siblings would never deliberately abandon their mom or her.

Even though they could not grant her leave, Jean's job was understanding of her situation. She had a lot of calls to and from the hospital and physicians. Some calls required talking to the doctor on speakerphone.

Caretaking often requires making and receiving numerous phone calls from hospitals, clinics, therapy, and more. One of the anxieties Jean experienced was that she never knew when someone on the medical team would return a phone call.

Jean confessed, "I was blessed to have this employer. I sat in a cubicle and had the type of job where I could work and still field the phone calls."

Jean talked about coping from a spiritual viewpoint. "I did a lot of praying. I cried to Jesus. I would not have made it if I did not have faith that God would take care of Mom. I prayed over her, especially when she was in pain, asking the Lord to please give the doctors wisdom to get her out of pain. Just to see her come out of the hospital after that kind of accident was a blessing in itself."

There was a silver lining to this tragedy. The night of Victoria's accident, friends of Jean's heard about the accident and showed up at the hospital. One of the guys, Raymond, came back the next day and offered to help Jean with transportation. He had just retired from the military, and Jean discovered in their conversations that he was going through a divorce. Instrumental in helping Jean get back and forth to the hospital every day, she came to rely on him emotionally as well. He was compassionate and helpful, and over time, their feelings grew.

Jean recounts a time when her company had a retreat about an hour away right after her mom had the accident. She had been spending nights at the hospital but was torn because the retreat was an important part of her job. Raymond offered to stay overnight with her mom at the hospital, so Jean went to the retreat while he took care of Victoria. Jean knew in her heart this was the man for her.

"Mom's accident was in September; she came home in December. I was still so focused on Mom; I did not think much about the future. On Christmas Day, the same month Mom came home, Ray proposed to me. I was stunned and stuttered, 'OK.' I have never regretted that decision. He helped me out so much and is kind and loving."

One thing Jean did not need to deal with was the legal issues. Victoria had made her eldest son her power of attorney. In addition, it was eventually determined that the school bus involved in the accident had turned on a green light, having not seen Victoria due to the sun. Her eldest son hired attorneys to represent her with the school bus's insurance company.

The other fortunate part of Victoria's tragic accident was that she had good health insurance with her job. Between her insurance and the legal settlement, they did not have to worry about major hospital bills.

Home

When it was time for Victoria to be released, there was another round of discussions between the siblings regarding their mom and if she should go to a nursing home. Jean stood up for her mom, and finally, Victoria was able to go back to her own home. It was a happy day when she could finally be in her familiar surroundings and sleep in her own bed.

While Jean was happy her mom was home, she knew that this was the end of her dream of going to Hawaii because her mom would require care in a different sort of way. Jean and Raymond now lived twenty-five miles away. It would be a longer drive to get to her mom's house before and after work each day.

Victoria's memory was different due to the brain contusions. She had to learn all over how to read and write. She could not remember large words and could not string sentences together. She would need to go for speech therapy at least three times a week. Raymond worked nights, so he took Victoria to therapy while Jean worked. They would put Jean on speakerphone to include her in Victoria's progress.

Victoria came home on a number of medications. Again, Jean put her creative mind to work. She bought a tackle box to sort the meds, and her mom learned what pills to take and when. Her mom tracked her medications. She also recorded what she ate as well as whom she talked to each day. It was also a good mental exercise for her.

Jean was resourceful. She had a book chock full of information on who to call and what resources were available.

She also did a lot of reading on medications, what they were for, and how long they should be taken. "People told me I missed my calling; I should have been in the medical field. I said no, I just like to read and learn."

Victoria used an electric wheelchair, which was fortunately covered by insurance. The local public transportation company had an option for handicapped mobility, so she could get around with the chair. As soon as she could, Victoria returned to serving as an election judge, riding her electric wheelchair down the street to the polling place.

Jean arranged for a housecleaner for Victoria, and had a caregiver come in for half days for several months.

Every evening, Jean would stop by her mom's house and make sure she had food to eat that night and the next day.

Jean got her a safety alert necklace. Every day at noon, the alert company called Victoria to make sure she was okay. Jean was first on the list to call in the event of an emergency. It gave them all peace of mind.

Victoria had been organized and meticulous with her banking and bills. But now, Jean needed to take over her mom's finances. As organized as her mom had been, it took a lot of research to figure out what needed paying and when, especially with Victoria's paycheck disruption. Her mom was unable to tell her if what Jean was doing was correct.

They were also concerned about her rent because it took a while to sort out the finances. Fortunately, the landlord was patient and flexible with the rent payments until the insurance money started arriving on a regular basis.

In spite of having help, Jean describes this time period as "absolutely exhausting." The caregiving took its toll on her health. Caregivers are usually taken by surprise at how much caring for another person takes its toll.

February brought joy as Jean and Raymond got married. Jean said, "I got a husband out of the deal, and I would not have made it without him."

A New Generation

Finally, things were calming down, and the family got into a rhythm. Jean and her husband visited Victoria periodically, and Victoria was getting on with her daily life. Married life was predictable and pleasant—for a short time.

One day, the phone rang, and it was Jean's oldest daughter Sheila calling from Hawaii. "Mom, I have a situation. I'm going to have a baby." Sheila had gotten pregnant while in college.

Sheila moved to Georgia with the baby's father where Alyssa was born. Jean was there for the birth where they quickly realized the relationship with the man was not going to work out. Jean brought her daughter and grandbaby to Minnesota when Alyssa was three days old.

They discussed if Sheila should return to school, and all agreed an education was critical. It was decided Sheila would return to school in Hawaii, and Jean and her husband agreed to keep Alyssa until their daughter got settled. When Alyssa was six months old, they brought her to Hawaii so she could live with her mom. It went well at first, but within six months, Alyssa developed asthma. It seemed Minnesota would be a better place for little Alyssa where she could get proper healthcare.

Jean and Raymond traveled to Hawaii where Jean scanned her "lost paradise." Knowing Jean was needed for her mom, the couple returned home, now a family of three. Little Alyssa thrived in Minnesota where the climate was much easier on her asthma.

Five years passed. Victoria had regular doctor's appointments, including an annual physical, and seemed to be doing well. She decided the alert button was an extra expense and not needed anymore. Jean lamented sarcastically, "My smart self said, 'Okay, she can send it back.'" That hasty decision would plague Jean.

Jean called her mom after work one day, and her mom did not answer. Jean stopped by her mom's home on the way home from work and rang her doorbell. No answer. Jean noticed something odd. Her mom's blinds were closed. Jean said, "Mom never kept lights on in the house. She opened up her blinds because that was 'God's light.'" She went home and asked her husband to go check on her mom on his way to work.

Raymond rang the bell but got no answer. On instinct, he decided to break the door open and found Jean's mom lying on the floor. He called the ambulance, and once again, Victoria was rushed to the hospital.

When Raymond called to give Jean the news that he had found Victoria lying on the floor, Jean's heart sank. Her precious mom may have laid there from noon until the evening when Raymond checked on her. Jean felt more caregiver guilt and more "What ifs?" and beating herself up for not forcing her way into the house.

When they arrived at the emergency room, the doctor said he hoped Victoria would pass quickly so that she would not have to suffer. Jean was horrified and told the doctor, "You do not know the God we know." She was hopeful her mom would get well and come home soon.

The doctor let them know Victoria had diabetes. Jean's mind flashed back to the time six years ago when the nurse nearly gave Victoria insulin. Was that a precursor to this situation? No, Jean shook her head. It was not possible.

Victoria's sugar level was down to 9 mg/dL. (A normal level is 100 to 125 mg/dL.) Diabetes did run in the family, but they had no idea Victoria had diabetes. Looking back, Jean remembered her mom had mentioned the week before that the back of her hand was black, but they assumed it was just bruising. Skin darkening can happen with diabetes.

Jean said she has learned to not only have one's glucose checked regularly but also the A1C level, which is the average glucose over three months.

With Victoria in the hospital the second time, her family asked if Jean would stay with her. Jean said, no, it was impossible this time. She was raising her granddaughter who still suffered from asthma, and Jean had developed her own health issues, including anxiety attacks. She was older now and had to manage her own series of medical appointments. "I had to get myself together," Jean emphatically stated.

The second day Victoria was in the hospital, the doctor said it was time to disconnect Victoria from life support and let her go. When the doctor left the room, the nurse said not to let them disconnect her because she was showing signs of life. When she talked to Victoria, she squeezed the nurse's hand.

Victoria's great-granddaughter came to visit her, and Victoria woke up and was alert for the day. She knew who the president was and how many grandkids she had. They had renewed hope.

Two weeks passed with Victoria on the ventilator. Two weeks in suspended animation. The family hung between life and what came next. Slowly, Victoria slipped back into her silent world. Later, they learned she had sepsis from the stool backing up into her abdomen, gangrene in her fingers, and other issues.

Jean said, "One thing I learned was to always check to see if they have a bag for stool for the patient. They collect urine, but they should also collect the stool."

They decided to start to clean mom's house out while the kids were all home. One of Victoria's sons opened a drawer by her bed and found a signed document stating she did not want to be on a ventilator. It also said she wanted to be cremated. The six kids read it and agreed it was indeed written by their mom, and they should abide by her wishes.

The hospital called a family meeting with the doctor. He explained the life Victoria would live if she remained alive on the ventilator.

With a catch in her throat, Jean said, "We had to decide if we wanted her to remain that way or disconnect her. It was agreed by all of the children to disconnect her. The doctor told us that it would not be long before she would pass after she was off of the ventilator. However, she lived a little more than two weeks."

And then, on her own, Victoria slipped into a blessed eternity. Victoria, who had been full of life and loved her family beyond measure, came to the end of her earthly life to pass on to see her Savior Jesus in Heaven, the "true paradise."

At first, after her mom died, Jean was not at peace. Why didn't they stay on top of her health? She always wondered if they had taken her mom to the doctor more often, would it have been any different? Victoria was only seventy-six when she died.

"I advise people to go to the doctor regularly and find out if there are health issues. I only wish I had done so with my mom."

Jean was thankful her mom did not suffer. She died peacefully. Had she lived, they would have likely had to remove her fingers, and Victoria would not have wanted to live that way.

The funeral was a memorial service at the church where Victoria and Raymond were members.

"It was a wonderful celebration," crowed Jean.

It was almost as though Raymond had lost his own mother. He had taken Victoria to many of the doctor's appointments, and he faithfully brought her to church. At the memorial service, church members came up to Raymond, thinking it was his mother who had died. Jean chuckles at this memory.

Advice

Jean, how would you advise other caregivers?

- I never found counseling for myself, but maybe I should have.
- Talk to someone while you are caregiving, even if it is not a family member. Take help where you can get it. If someone needs to be at the hospital, get help. Do not be there yourself every single day.
- Talk to your higher power if you have one. If you do not have one, find one.
- Do not take the first response from the professionals as final. Research and learn as much as you can.

Author's Reflections

Jean said her mom's health problems in Gary were not related to her race; they were related to poverty. Later, they were a result of aging.

When her mom was in the hospital in Minnesota Jean noted, "The hospital staff treated my mom well. However, she often had a family member with her, and if there were to be a problem, I would not have let Mom be mistreated. The whole family would advocate for her."

Jean describes herself as persistent, faithful, and dedicated. I know when she goes to her heavenly paradise, she will hear the words of Jesus: *"Well done, good and faithful servant."* (Matthew 25:21).

Healthcare Disparity

Indeed, healthcare disparities do exist, and much work remains to be done. The pandemic of 2020 has magnified the need to lift people out of poverty and hopelessness. We can all learn lessons from Jean about diligence, advocating for our own, and family love. We can also educate ourselves and advocate for equality for healthcare for all people. The following information is in the public domain from U.S. Government data.

The *2019 National Healthcare Quality and Disparities Report* from the Agency for Healthcare Research and Quality shows the progress and opportunities for improving healthcare quality and reducing healthcare disparities.

Disparities: Overall, some disparities were getting smaller from 2000 through 2016-2018, but disparities persist and some even worsened, especially for poor and uninsured populations in all priority areas.

Racial and ethnic disparities vary by group:

- For about 40% of quality measures, Blacks (82 of 202) and American Indians and Alaska Natives (47 of 116) received worse care than Whites. For more than one-third of quality measures, Hispanics (61 of 177) received worse care than Whites.
- For nearly 30% of quality measures, Asians (52 of 185) received worse care than Whites, but Asians received better care than Whites for nearly one-third (56 of 185) of quality measures.
- Poor is defined as having family income below 100% of the federal poverty level.

Disparities vary by residence location:

- For one-third of quality measures, Native Hawaiians/Pacific Islanders (24 of 72) received worse care than Whites.
- For nearly a quarter (24 of 102) of quality measures, residents of large central metropolitan areas received worse care than residents of large fringe metropolitan areas.
- For one-third of quality measures, residents of micropolitan and noncore areas received worse care than residents of large fringe metropolitan areas.
- For a little less than 20% of quality measures, medium and small metropolitan residents received worse care than residents of large fringe metropolitan areas.[4]

Chapter 6
Finding Purpose in Pain

*"The two most important days in your life are
the day you were born, and
the day you find out why."*
– Mark Twain

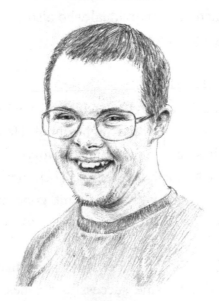

Introduction

Diana and Greg had no reason to think their life would take a heartbreaking curve. They married in their twenties, ran a successful business, and soon added a daughter to their family. Their families lived close by, and together, they celebrated the joys of parenthood.

No one could have predicted what came next. Call it a one-two punch. Despair and fear.

Many families would not survive this situation with their marriage intact. Others would choose institutional solutions, and there is no judgment here about those decisions. Families must determine the best course of action when life does not turn out as hoped and planned. But I think you will discover through this story, as I did, how one family found meaning through suffering and found and implemented unique solutions. At the end, you will meet an incredible individual who also found meaning and purpose through this family's story.

The Best of Plans

It was 1982 in an idyllic small town where high school sweethearts parted ways after high school. He finished college and started a business. She attended two years of college and was on her way to finish her degree. They met again, and Greg was once more smitten with the vibrant, good-natured Diana.

"Stay here. We will get married and run the business together," he cajoled.

Diana said, "I bought it hook, line, and sinker!"

They married, became successful business owners, and a beautiful baby girl named Mindy followed. She had been born by cesarean section weighing in at a healthy nine pounds four ounces.

While life was not perfect, the future looked bright for the young family. They decided to have a second child. As planned, within two years of Mindy arriving on the scene, Diana and Greg were expecting their second child. Still in their twenties, they had no reason to believe this pregnancy would not go as well as the first.

The pregnancy moved along with no problems—until the end. During an ultrasound, the physician was having trouble determining Diana's due date.

He murmured, "We usually measure the due date of the fetus by the femur bone. This baby's femur bone is a little longer than we would expect. Kids with Down syndrome have a longer femur leg bone than the tibia, we will check it again at the next ultrasound." However, after three ultrasounds, they did not see any other unusual problems, and assumed the longer femur bone was a harmless irregularity.

Diana wanted to have this second baby naturally instead of cesarean. The decision was made to induce her. They drove to the small local community hospital at 7:00 a.m. where she was given the medication to start labor. Labor progressed, but Diana struggled to push out this baby.

Knowing the size of Mindy, the doctor wondered if they should continue or proceed with a cesarean birth. They decided to try a little longer.

At 4:09 p.m., the birth was imminent, so the doctor reached in, grabbed the baby by the fat on the back of the neck, and pulled. Out came baby number two with a broken collar bone (not all that rare with the soft bones), weighing in at ten pounds three ounces.

They had a baby boy and named him Tyler.

The first couple of weeks were different from their first weeks with Mindy. Tyler would not nurse. He would try so hard, but then he would fall asleep. He just did not have the muscle tone to suck properly. Diana consulted an obstetric nurse who helped her figure out how to feed Tyler. Still, things did not seem quite right.

When Tyler was three months old, he developed a bad cold. It turned out to be pneumonia, and the rural doctors could not figure out why he did not get better. Over a period of a couple of months, they sought additional treatments. Finally, the local doctor recommended they see a specialist in a larger town about thirty miles away. There, they tested him for cystic fibrosis. To the relief of the anxious parents, the test came back negative.

Dual Diagnosis

But their anxiety was not quelled for long. The doctor said, "We need to test Tyler for Down syndrome."

Diana groaned. "You could have punched Greg and me in the gut."

The doctor had a brother with Down syndrome, so he recognized the signs. It was 1991, and all genetic tests were sent to the Mayo Clinic. It would take ten days to get the results.

"A horrific ten days," fretted Diana.

Meanwhile, Tyler was still sick with pneumonia.

Finally, the phone rang. It was the doctor. The results were in.

"I'm sorry to let you know the test came back positive. Tyler has Down syndrome."

The stunned parents did not know what to say.

> Down syndrome, also known as trisomy 21, is a genetic disorder caused by the presence of all or part of a third copy of chromosome 21.

Events started clicking into place: the longer femur, an extra roll of fat on the neck, the high birth weight, and poor muscle control were all common traits of Down syndrome. One reason they did not suspect Down syndrome was because Tyler did not have the distinct features of Down syndrome other than Brushfield's spots in his eyes.

> Brushfield's spots are little white slightly elevated spots on the surface of the iris and arranged in a ring around the pupil. They can be found in all children but are more common in people with Down syndrome.

The physician was helpful, even though he personally did not have a lot of experience with people with disabilities. He gave Diana and Greg time to let the diagnosis sink in.

Then he said, "This life will be hard for you, but for Tyler, every day is going to be like Christmas. He will not be aware of the bad things in the world. He won't be aware of what is frightening. He will only be aware of events that are pleasing and fun to him."

Diana acknowledged that this was comforting and often true. "However, every day is not quite like Christmas for Tyler. Since he is minimally verbal, it is hard to know what he is thinking or what he wants when he is frustrated."

Because Tyler was still sick, the doctor recommended they go to the children's hospital in Minneapolis several hours drive away. They brought Tyler home, knowing they would need time to adjust to the Down syndrome diagnosis. The appointment could wait a couple of days.

But time was not on their side. That same night, two weeks before Christmas, baby Tyler had a breathing crisis. The family rushed to the nearby satellite clinic where they diagnosed him with atelectasis in his lungs. It had been coming on for a couple of months. They stabilized Tyler and told the family to take him to the children's hospital immediately.

> Atelectasis is a complete or partial collapse of either the entire lung or a lobe of the lung. The tiny air sacs within the lung become deflated or are filled with fluid.

The young family rushed to the children's hospital in the middle of the night. They took Tyler into the emergency room and treatment started immediately. This was a teaching hospital, and many people were interested in Tyler's situation. Diana and Greg had to keep telling their story over and over.

After a lengthy evaluation, a new doctor came into their room. He was a pediatric oncologist who broke more bad news to Diana and Greg. "Tyler is in a pre-leukemia state. He will develop leukemia; we just do not know when. It could be weeks, months—but it will happen."

It was a double whammy. One day, they learned their precious son had Down syndrome, and the next day, they were told he would develop leukemia. Overnight, their world spun upside down.

There was no internet back then; learning came from other people and books. They discovered that kids with Down syndrome either have heart problems or develop leukemia. Fortunately, Tyler did not have heart problems.

Before long, they learned Tyler had Acute Myeloid Leukemia (AML).

> AML starts in the bone marrow (the soft inner part of certain bones where new blood cells are made) and quickly moves into the blood. It can also spread to other parts of the body.

Tyler was treated for his lung problems at the children's hospital, and further evaluations for his cancer took place. Three days before Christmas, Tyler was able to go home. The stunned family spent Christmas with family, sad, scared, and worried. "But we did our best to show Mindy our family would be okay," admitted Diana.

Large bone marrow cells fragment off into smaller cells called platelets. Platelets clump up and control bleeding. Tyler's bone marrow struggled to make good blood platelets; they would die off as soon as the fragments broke off. Weekly blood draws were taken at the local rural hospital, and when they got the results, Diana called the oncologist in the city to report the blood counts. Everyone anxiously watched the counts because when his counts reached a certain point, Tyler would start getting chemotherapy.

Meanwhile, Mindy, who was three when her brother was born, turned four when Tyler started his cancer treatments. She spent a lot of time with her grandparents, aunt, uncle, and cousins while Greg and Diana focused on keeping their business going and Tyler's duo medical diagnosis.

Finally, Tyler's platelets and hemoglobin were low enough to begin the chemotherapy. They headed to the children's hospital. In lieu of constant blood draws or inserting medication in his veins, Tyler had a Hickman catheter coming out of his chest. One line was for blood transfusions and one for medicine.

> A Hickman line is a central venous catheter most often used for the administration of chemotherapy or other medications as well as for the withdrawal of blood for analysis.

Then came the first bone marrow biopsy. Diana shuddered even all of these years later when she shared, "With a needle as big as a straw, they extracted the bone marrow out of little hip bones." Tyler was ten months old when they started the treatment.

Diana and Greg have a strong Catholic faith, and a local priest ministered to them at the hospital. He warned them, "A family with a disabled or terminally ill child is at risk. Many people in your situation get a divorce. You need to take care of yourselves and your relationship."

The young couple clung to each other, and divorce seemed like a far-off possibility. But life got more complicated and increasingly difficult, and their relationship was challenged in ways they could not imagine in those early days.

In spite of her faith, Diana did not go to church for three months. "I was so angry. What did I ever do to deserve this? Why God? Why me? Why Tyler? Why us? People would say, 'Tyler needed special parents,' or 'God picked you.' At the time, I just could not see the rationale for this situation."

Then Diana paused and took a deep breath. "Now I know why…"

The "why" was a long time coming. But let us go back to baby Tyler. At this point, they did not know if Tyler would live to see his first birthday, and if he did survive, they did not know what his quality of life would be.

Treatment Protocol

Tyler had always been unique. His birth was unique, his first few months were different, and his Down syndrome was not typical in many ways. Because he was so unique, everyone at the hospital wanted to learn from Tyler. His parents were asked to give assent to a clinical trial treatment protocol.

A clinical trial is a research study that assigns a subject to a particular treatment arm. The scientists collect data to learn how effective the treatment looks. The protocol is a document that describes how a clinical trial will be conducted. It is designed to ensure the safety of the trial subject, and the results are based on data collection. A patient needs to consent to the protocol, and if they cannot consent, a patient or legal representative can "assent" to the treatment.

The whole medical team knew Tyler was put on the treatment protocol, and they anxiously watched and waited to see how Tyler would react. Diana and Greg became the go-to parents on the pediatric oncology wing.

The first step in the protocol was the chemotherapy regime. It was scheduled for one week a month for seven continuous days at the children's hospital. The chemo drug (which Diana described as "poison") would be pumped into Tyler's Hickman catheter. After the week was over, they would head back home to their business and daughter.

Again, once a week, Tyler would have blood work done at the local hospital. His counts fell, which was "good" because it meant the chemo was working. Unfortunately, however, it left Tyler vulnerable to illness. Sometimes, he would need a platelet transfusion, and because the local hospital did not have the capability of transfusing an infant, back to the city they headed.

There was only a twenty percent chance their sweet baby boy would survive. But twenty percent was better than zero, and they were committed to beating the odds.

Nine rounds of chemo. Nine months of trips to the city through rain or snow. Then there were extra drives for transfusions when needed.

Slowly, the bone marrow started to recover.

Diana reported, "The worst part about it all, after nine months of chemo, was Tyler reached a point in the protocol where the computer randomizes children to one of two routines: Treatment Arm One, two rounds of an intense chemo treatment with no recovery time. Treatment Arm Two was to go to the U of MN for a bone marrow transplant. This was 1992, and while the U of MN was a leader in bone marrow transplantation, they were fairly new as a standard course of treatment.

They met with one of the physicians at the Bone Marrow Transplant Unit at the U of MN. The physician looked at Tyler and asked, "Does Tyler have Down syndrome?" Diana said that he did. The doctor said she would be right back.

Diana lost it, knowing her heart would break if she got any more bad news. She and Greg sat in the room, bracing for the report, and praying for a glimmer of hope.

The doctor walked briskly into the room. "I have good news for you," explained the doctor. "The U of MN just finished a study on babies who have Down syndrome AML. The study has not been released to the public, but the findings indicate when the children take the intensive care route, their chances of survival are 80 percent!"

Diana said, "We felt like a miracle happened in that chair. We felt like God was on our side."

There is so much more to this story but suffice it to say that this was an emotional and spiritual turning point for the family.

Tyler was taken off the initial clinical trial and placed on this new intensive chemotherapy treatment for children with Down syndrome. The bone marrow transplant was now not an option.

Not that the intensive chemo was easy. Between the harshness of the chemo and continuous infections, they feared Tyler might not make it. A normal white blood cell count is between 4,000 and 11,000 per microliter of blood—Tyler's dropped to 100. Blood and lung infections made Tyler sicker and sicker. Most children who die during the treatment die from infections, a thought the worried parents tried to push out of their minds.

We Need a Miracle

The anxious family gathered by Tyler's bedside. One night, Greg, Diana, and both of their moms were at the hospital. Diana did not want to leave her son's bedside.

"Diana, you have to get some rest," both moms advised.

Diana had barely slept for the past three days. She said, "I was tearful, on edge, shaky. And crabby!"

The hospital had apartments connected to the hospital and available to patient's families. While it was only six halls down, Diana was fearful something would happen if she left Tyler's side.

"I will stay right by his side. You go sleep for a few hours," offered Greg.

In her heart, Diana knew they were right. She had to sleep. Diana and her mom headed back to the room to rest. Diana took a long hot shower, put on her pajamas, and curled up in a big chair, still certain she would not be able to sleep. Her eyes fluttered shut.

The hotel phone jangled loudly. Diana jerked awake.

It was Greg. "You need to come now."

Diana threw her clothes back on, and the two women ran down the halls.

Greg's mom was sitting in a rocking chair with Tyler. The nurse had just taken his temperature, which had climbed to 105 degrees F. The family was quiet other than their murmured prayers. They knew God was with them, but would he touch little Tyler with His healing hand? Or would they be preparing for a funeral in a couple of days?

The doctor came in and spoke in a compassionate but matter-of-fact way. "Tyler might not make it through the night. I just want you to be prepared."

The family nodded, solemn and tearful.

Greg's mom kept rocking Tyler. She let out a little sigh, reached down to kiss her grandson's forehead, and a puzzled look crossed across her face.

She gasped. "Quick, call the nurse!"

Three heads snapped up, and Diana, with adrenalin overrunning her exhaustion, pushed the nurse call button.

When the nurse came in, Greg's mom inhaled, and in one quick breath, she said, "You need to take his temperature because he feels really cool."

Tyler's temperature was normal. His blood pressure was normal. A miracle had occurred right there in the hospital room.

Tyler got better, and he kept improving. The intensive chemotherapy arm was discontinued, and instead, a round of oral pills was described. They could crush the pills, mixing them with applesauce and other soft foods.

The doctors were slow to say Tyler was in remission. He continued to have bone marrow aspirations, which is bone marrow removed by a needle out of the pelvic bones. Diana still winces at the thought of that large needle being inserted into her son's pelvis. But the news was good. There were fewer and fewer immature cells.

Christmas was coming around again. What a year it had been! Finally, the doctor could say with confidence that Tyler was in remission! The whole family had a huge celebration.

After the final dose of chemotherapy, Tyler never had to have chemo again.

During and after his hospital stays, Tyler had occupational and physical therapy. But now at one-and-a-half years old, they could concentrate on assessing and treating the effects of Down syndrome.

The therapies focused on Tyler's needs. He learned to drink from a cup, crawl, and sit up. Muscles were slowly strengthened, and motor skills developed. Life did not return to "normal," but they started on the path to a "new normal."

Diana and Greg spent as much time as they could with Mindy. Siblings of children with disabilities have their own needs.

Diana said, "We always made an extra effort to not burden Mindy with Tyler's disability. We let her be in every sport she could be in. We supported her in every endeavor. We wanted to make sure our whole life was not just about her brother."

The "new normal" included support from family members. The schools had excellent services and provided special education teachers. Time passed as the family of four settled into a routine, sometimes with bumps, but together.

The Answer to "Why?"

Diana and Greg's faith in God was slowly but surely restored. Over time, the answer to the questions, "Why God?

Why us?" came to Diana.

She said, "This happened because God said, 'I need your help, Diana and Greg. I need you to go out there and teach others that individuals with disabilities are people too. They can have a life, can be fulfilled, but maybe in a different way. Keep pushing your message. Keep teaching people.'

"Now I know why God picked us. Because we have pushed the boundaries. When there were obstacles, we found a way to overcome. In every situation, we had to find a way to have inclusion for Tyler. We taught people who Tyler is and why."

Diana and Greg started a fund for kids with cancer named after their son, and they continue to raise money for other families suffering from cancer. Over forty-three kids in their local area have been able to fight cancer with a $2,000 gift.

One example of Diana and Greg's unique problem-solving was to create "The Player of the Game." At every home game for all of the different sports in their school, they would pick an athlete who was "The Player of the Game." Tyler would get his picture taken with that student, and Diana and Greg would donate $25 to Tyler's cancer fund in the athlete's name. The message was "It was okay. Do not be afraid of him. Tyler is a young person just like you. He wants dreams and needs the same things you do."

An emotional Diana continues the story. "Tyler made it through high school. On his graduation day in their small community, there was to be no clapping until the entire student body received their diplomas. But as Tyler crossed the stage, spontaneous clapping broke out throughout the entire auditorium. We knew we had made a difference. Tyler's life made a difference."

Diana then smiled. "Tyler just went to his ten-year class reunion. His dad took him. (Who wants their mom at their class reunion?) The kids were still accepting, welcoming, and enthusiastically greeted him."

Tyler, All Grown Up

Graduation was over, and Tyler's classmates were going to college or getting married and starting their own families. Diana and Greg knew Tyler needed his own life, and they needed a life for themselves after all of these years.

Another thought played in the back of their minds as a major source of stress for parents of disabled children loomed large: what happens when the parents can no longer care for the child? What will happen to Tyler, assuming he outlives his parents?

Diana and Greg talked and re-talked about different options. Diana did a lot of the research.

By this time, Mindy had graduated from college. She was planning a wedding and had launched her own career. Diana and Greg did not want to burden Mindy with her brother's care—being a caregiver 24/7 is hard work. Alternative arrangements had to be made.

They made certain all of the legal paperwork was in place as they started searching for solutions. No obstacle was too great for this resilient family.

While a group home is the answer for some families, Diana and Greg knew this setting would not work for Tyler. In a typical group home, the staff comes and goes, and there are different personalities to get used to. Tyler did not deal well with change, so each new day would be a struggle for him in a group home.

Diana met with a community group of moms who also had kids with disabilities. Together, they supported each other and brainstormed ideas. They also worked with Tyler's social worker who connected them with Lutheran Social Service (LSS). With LSS, Diana and Greg developed the idea of a "Reverse Host Home."

Instead of placing Tyler in a group home, what if Tyler had a home and a "host parent" lived with him? Could they build or find such a house? Would anyone be willing to live in this situation? Would Tyler adjust?

Their initial plan was to build a house and find a caregiver to live in the house. It would need to be someone who loved and appreciated people with disabilities and would be willing to be on call twenty-four hours a day, seven days a week.

The idea to build a house was not working out. As they explored alternatives, a house a half a mile down the road from Diana and Greg's home went up for sale. This seemed like a workable solution. The house needed renovation, so the whole family, including Tyler, went to work. Tyler cleaned, painted, and helped pick out furnishings.

Next was to find the "host parent." Diana's niece was unemployed and living with her parents. She agreed to stay until they found someone permanent.

It was an anxious time for the family, especially Diana. Like all moms, she knew it was time to launch her baby bird out of the nest, but would it really work out? Could her "baby"—the one they nursed through cancer, struggled with to teach the basics of self-care, and labored with through twelve grades of school— survive without her by his side? He was barely verbal and needed help with nearly all his daily living tasks. What *would* he do without Mom and Dad by his side?

Who among us parents do not worry when our son or daughter goes off to college or is on their own for the first time? Imagine that plus having a child with many challenges.

Finally, it was moving day. The whole family was there. "It was a huge day," Diana exclaimed. She had been crying for weeks, happy tears as well as stressful tears.

When morning dawned, they got up, had a family breakfast, and finished loading the last of Tyler's stuff. Soon—maybe too soon for Mom and Dad—everything was loaded.

Diana, Greg, Mindy, and her husband, Peter, were all in the kitchen, crying and holding onto each other. Was this the right next step? Had they made a mistake? Where was Tyler—hiding in his room?

No. Tyler was in the car waiting, ready to go. He was not at all anxious like the rest of the family. He was excited!

Diana laughed. "There was not a better indication from God we were doing the right thing. Even though we had gone over the story fifteen times, we were never sure if he understood. But Tyler was ready to go!"

The baby bird was ready to leave the nest. The parents, like all of us, were both ready and apprehensive.

To make the situation more affordable, they had searched for another young man to live in the house. They found Michael who also had Down syndrome and was about Tyler's age. Michael had tragically lost both of his parents, leaving the siblings with no plan for his care. They too were searching for a solution, so it was decided that Michael and Tyler would become roommates.

Diana reported, "After moving into his own home, Tyler grew up and became a different person. He understands Mom and Dad have a life. When he comes to visit us for a weekend, we always plan to bring him home after the evening meal. About 3:00, Tyler says, 'Home.' He wants to be at his house just like any other normal person his age."

Diana's niece stayed for a year-and-a-half. She helped them through the transition, and they all learned a lot in that time. When her niece was ready to move on with her life, they looked for a full-time caregiver. By God's provision, they were blessed when Diana's friend Angie gladly took on the responsibility. Angie, Tyler, and Michael have made the house a home for four years now.

When Angie wants to take a vacation, Diana and Greg take Tyler home or pay for a caregiver from the community. Michael's siblings oversee his care and plan for him as needed.

Diana, Greg, Mindy, Peter, Tyler, Michael, and Angie were special guests at am LSS event last year where over one-thousand people were in attendance. Tyler, Michael, and Angie were asked to stand and be recognized. The three had huge smiles on their faces as the audience applauded.

"My heart melted; we were so proud!" crowed Diana.

Diana and Greg have done many speaking engagements, educating people, and sharing their story.

As the boys settled into their new home, Diana and Greg sought other ways to provide opportunities for the boys and others with disabilities. Working through the Disabled Adult Child (DAC) County Program, they started "North of Ordinary," a business for people with disabilities. The workers perform tasks such as cleaning and sorting inventory and receive a wage. At first, Angie would go with Tyler and Michael to work at North of Ordinary, but now, the boys independently take a bus. They are proud of the work they do, and the families know they have a purpose in their lives.

Reflections

Diana reflected, "In our life, we have been touched by the grace of God in many, many ways. In Tyler's schooling, we were so blessed, and now, he has this opportunity to live in his own home. God had it all laid out. We just had to go down the road. It is amazing how it all fell together. We just feel the grace of God helped us do all those things."

If Tyler still lived at home, Diana and Greg would not have a life as a couple. Caring for another person twenty-four hours a day, seven days a week is so hard on a relationship. Now, they are able to concentrate on the family business, entertain in their home, and go on vacation without the constant challenge of caregiving.

Mindy grew up to be a loving and giving sister. She and Tyler are close siblings, and they love each other beyond measure. Mindy shares "our" story through her work and has made documentaries about her brother. She and Peter have their own life in a different state but stay in close contact with their families.

Tyler turned twenty-nine in May 2020. He is starting to show heart problems from some of the drugs he had to treat his cancer, but overall, he is doing well.

In the beginning when people told Diana and Greg, "God hand-picked you," it made them angry. Why would God pick them? But now, they do believe God picked them to be the parents of Tyler, to share their story, and to teach others about the beauty of their child with disabilities.

Diana also reflects on the priest's warning about their marriage. They recently celebrated their thirty-fifth anniversary, but she acknowledges there were times this took nothing but hard work and grit.

"Three years into it, ten years into it, even thirty-five years into it, you have to take care of yourself. If the caregiver does not take care of him or herself, the caregiver will implode. And if Greg and I had not taken care of each other, we would have been divorced. It is so difficult."

Advice

Diana, what advice do you have for other parents of a child with disabilities?

- Set aside time to care for yourself, your marriage, and others in your family.
- Do not be so hard on yourself on the really, really hard days. Get through the moment, and then try to find a way to get through the next moment.
- Love unconditionally, even though you will have people in your life who do not understand and are cruel and just plain rude.
- Take every opportunity you can to be a teachable moment to others. Do not let it pass by and then wish you would have said something. It makes a difference, even if it is one person at a time.

- Share the joy of your child but share the hard moments too. Let people know when you need a hand, just a hug, or a moment to breathe. People want to help, but we need to make sure to accept it.
- You are blessed because you have been given a gift from God. Use your life to teach others about compassion and acceptance. It is okay to be different, and God loves us all!

Angie's View

This story would not be complete without Angie's viewpoint, the Reverse Home Host. She reflects on why she took this position and describes how she manages the job, which is her entire lifestyle.

Of note is the fact that Angie did not have any special training before she took on the position. The skills she has are a willingness to care for others, to learn, and to dedicate her life to caregiving for these two precious young men.

How did you decide to become the Reverse Home Host?

Becoming a host was a "fluke." As a young person, I worked in healthcare, including nursing homes. I then spent seventeen years at a private for-profit college working in administration and records management. The job was fast-paced and stressful. However, I enjoyed it for the most part at the time. I am a caring person at heart, and eventually, I felt a change was needed.

My daughter lived in our hometown a couple of hours away. "Mom, why don't you move back up here? We could hang out more and do things together," she pleaded.

After a lot of soul-searching, I quit my job, sold my house, and accepted an administrative job in my hometown. Before I knew it, I was packed up and headed to a new life.

The new job was pleasant enough. But the pace was slow, and I took a large pay cut. I was also in culture shock, having moved from a large metropolitan area back to a small town.

"Had I made a mistake?" I asked myself.

A year passed. It was another slow workday, and I glanced at my email when a message from my sister caught my eye. She worked for a friend of ours who was looking for a live-in caregiver for her son, Tyler, and his roommate. Might I be able to recommend someone for the job? I said to send me the job description.

I read the information about the position with interest. It was a paid position. The "host" would live in the house with two young men with Down syndrome. I was intrigued by the idea and called Diana, and we met to chat about the job. At first, Diana thought I was there to help her find the right person.

Next thing I know, I am in a conference room with Diana, her husband Greg, siblings of the other young man, and LSS, who oversees the Reverse Home Host Program. Diana told me about Tyler's needs. The other family told me about their brother Michael whose parents had both died within months of each other. The "conference" had turned into a job interview.

LSS would have to approve the host, and an adult foster care license through the county is required. LSS said I would hear back from their human resources department about the position.

As I walked out of the room, I knew I was qualified and could obtain the licensure needed. It sounded like a perfect fit, but would they accept me?

I waited to hear from the team, but no call came. I thought, *maybe they did not want me?* I waited. I hoped.

I finally picked up the phone and called LSS.

The representative apologized exclaiming, "I am so sorry! I got busy and forgot to call you back. The families wanted you before you even left the room!"

I let out my breath, not even realizing I had been holding it.

And that began my path to the biggest challenge and adventure of my life!

What are your responsibilities?

I obtained my license for adult foster care through the county. There had been another caretaker at the home for a year-and-a-half before I came, and when I started, the home licensing process began all over. Several county workers came to look at the house, including the fire marshal. The only issue they identified was the wood-burning fireplace had to have a lock and screen.

I care for the young men twenty-four hours a day, seven days a week. Each one has different needs. For example, Tyler needs more help with Activities of Daily Living (ADLs). I "mirror" what he should do, making motions to brush my teeth or apply deodorant. He mirrors back and does the action.

I do all of the clothes washing for Tyler, and he folds his washcloths, socks, and underwear. We hang up his t-shirts together. He does an excellent job with vacuuming; he picks up or moves everything on the floor, including plants, tables, shoes, or whatever is in his way.

Michael has more ability to do his own ADLs. He can wash and dry his own clothes, and he cleans the bathrooms. I need to supervise his computer time to ensure what he is watching is appropriate.

I clean, supervise, organize the kitchen, and do most of the cooking. The guys can do little things with cooking, like heating up breakfast sandwiches in the microwave or finding snacks, and they are both able to eat on their own.

The guys look at the grocery ads and make a list of what they want to eat for the week. As they do not know what we have at home, I pare down the list so that we only get what we need. We all go grocery shopping, and they help look for groceries. I will tell Tyler to look for green beans, and he picks out green beans. With Michael, I can be more specific and say, "Look for French cut green beans." He understands the difference in types of food.

We go on other outings in the community, much like a mom would go on with a twelve-year-old. We eat out, go to movies, and do our banking together. People in the community know us and are accepting of the guys. We also work in the garden together.

Neither young man can be without supervision. I can go out and mow the lawn, but I check in to make sure they are doing okay. Otherwise, I do not leave the property without them going with me or having another caregiver come in.

I administer their medications daily, documenting that and their daily activities, their daily interactions with people, and any behavior or health items they had for that day.

LSS has directors/coordinators specifically assigned to host homes. We have a great partnership. We talk about what is happening, and my coordinator advises me when I have questions. I have online trainings through LSS that the county accepts as equal to trainings they require in-person. They have been wonderful to work with this whole time.

What challenges have you faced, and how have you overcome them?

This job can be challenging, but not as challenging as being in a corporate setting.

I need to watch how I word requests. I have learned not to use "No," "You can't do that," or "Don't go there." Those words are a trigger for both guys, much like many of us. Instead, I rephrase my words or redirect their attention, and I never talk down to them.

Tyler in particular does not like to be told no. "Don't do this" or "You can't do that" causes him to get angry, and sometimes, that anger is expressed in a physical way. In the last six months, he has become more oppositional.

This is being written during the COVID-19 quarantine, so you can imagine how the shutdown affects people who do not have the ability to understand what is going on.

Tyler is not too verbal, but I can tell when he is getting agitated because he blinks his eyes more and uses hand gestures. When I see these behaviors start, I change my approach or redirect his attention. He especially likes Disney shows and Star Wars, so I will put those on for him to watch. In addition, the medical team is experimenting with different medications to address negative behaviors.

The other major challenge is time. Tyler does not like to go to bed at night and getting up in the morning is a challenge. I have tried to rephrase and restate, "Tyler, it is bedtime" in many different ways. Sometimes, it is 2:30 or 3:00 a.m. when he goes to sleep, but then he has to be up for work the next day. He has not worked much due to the fact that he does not get up in time to go. We did work with his workplace to get him to start later (11:30 a.m.), but sometimes, he still misses work because he does not get ready on time.

There are times I have nearly missed a personal appointment, such as seeing the dentist, because Tyler would not get up on time. I have to be prepared for a last-minute change or call and have someone come in and stay with him while I go to my appointment.

Michael keeps more regular hours. The bus picks him up for work at 9:30 a.m., and he is ready to go.

I am a problem solver. Tyler has his own sign language, but after two-and-a-half years, I still cannot clearly understand what he is trying to say. He can write, and he can read and understand quite a bit.

Michael is verbal, but he is also difficult to understand. Michael can write and spell several words, enough so I can usually decipher what he is saying. Sometimes, he will draw pictures to get his point out. When I do not understand what Michael wants, I let him know. He gets frustrated, but he does not get angry.

We keep active, gardening, working on the lawn, playing with bean bags, and more. We like to keep moving.

Do you have set time off or vacation days?

I do not have a set schedule of time off, but I do have respite time. Diana and Greg take Tyler a minimum of two weekends a month. Michael's family does not take him often. My sister has taken classes and is licensed in adult foster care so she can stay with the guys. For example, if it is just Michael, she will come and stay overnight. My daughter is also a licensed caregiver and can help out when needed.

I have taken a week-long vacation a couple of times since I started.

I wish more people would be licensed for respite care for adults. There is such a need, and this type of arrangement is starting to catch on.

What would you recommend for other caregivers in this situation?

First, patience is so important. Sometimes, I need to separate everyone into different rooms. If I get to the "end of my rope," I will go sit outside so I can catch my breath.

Second, realize your timing is not their timing. Your urgency is not their urgency. They just may not be ready to move. Start getting ready early. If there is a time when everyone is ready right at the same time, it is amazing!

Caregivers need to be prepared to not have time to themselves when there are no other outlets such as work, or families cannot take them. Respite persons are difficult to find. I have identified activities for the guys to do on their own so I can take a break in the backyard or in my room when alone time is needed.

In conclusion, Angie told me she is quite attached to both of the young men; they are like her kids. "This is the dream job I never knew I wanted."

It is easy to see why Diana calls Angie "my angel."

Author Reflections

Caretakers of parents or other adults have challenges and often experience heartbreak. Generally, however, there is an end, sad though that may be. Parents of children with disabilities know the end of the relationship may be their own demise; the child may outlive the parents. This brings a whole new set of challenges. Will the parent spend the rest of their life caring for the child? What will happen to the child when the parent dies?

The story of Tyler's family is sad yet hopeful, as it demonstrates the ability to identify solutions to these pressing problems. If you would like more information on finding or establishing a reverse host house, Lutheran Social Services of Minneapolis may serve as a resource.

Conclusion

Writing others' stories is a privilege. Learning about their lives and caregiving journeys has enhanced my respect for humanity. They remind me of the good in this world. I hope you were not only entertained but also felt their pain and joy and challenges and successes. There are so many lessons we can learn as present and future caregivers. While these stories only represent six families, they give us a picture of unselfishness and resilience.

Did I have any big revelations of human nature? Where there unique characteristics among these caregivers? I could write another book analyzing their personalities, love, fears, and determined natures, but the stories can speak for themselves. I am respectful of the incredible resilience and creativity it takes to be a successful caregiver.

Appendix 3 is a list of questions to be used by book clubs, caregiving groups, or others wishing to explore the "how" and "why" caregivers behave as they do. When providing an endorsement,

Merrill Kindall, retired pastor, stated, "*Remarkable Caregiving* would have been a must reading for my Stephen Caregivers Ministry at our previous church. I will personally make known my recommendation to them and previous congregations."

My hope is that *Remarkable Caregiving* will bring awareness, hope and empowerment to individuals and groups as we care for our family and friends.

Appendix 1
Financial and Legal Review

> Not intended to replace the financial or legal advice of professionals.

When you have a loved one needing extra care, a whole lot of heartache can be saved by planning ahead. Whether you are an offspring caring for parent, a parent caring for a disabled child, or a spouse, sibling, or other close family member, ensuring the proper paperwork is in place can save a whole lot of heartache.

This appendix contains a list of suggestions for families to review. These have been gathered from various resources and my personal experiences.

Finances and Documents

Advisors: Make a list of your loved one's advisors, both the companies and any names available:

- Attorney
- Financial Advisor
- Insurance Agent(s): Home, Vehicles, Life Insurance, and Long-term Care

Assets: Do they own pensions, individual retirement accounts (IRAs), stocks, bonds, etc. If so, what organizations are they through, and how are those assets managed?

Banking: Where does your loved one bank? Do they have a safety deposit box, and if yes, where is the key?

Bills: What bills do they have? Are any of them paid automatically or electronically? How much is their house payment, association dues, or rent?

Funeral or Memorial Service: What will happen when they die? Do they have cremation, burial, or funeral plans? If so, do you know where the paperwork can be found?

If they do not have a plan in place, you may want to help them purchase one, as it is the one asset that can be excluded when applying for Medical Assistance/Medicaid.

Social Security: Do they receive Social Security? How much, and when does it come?

Important Documents: Where does your love one store copies of important papers? Are the copies paper or electronic? Can you find documents such as birth certificates, house and vehicle titles, and marriage or divorce certificates? How about green cards or proof of citizenship?

Passwords: Does your loved one have a password list, paper or electronic? Can you access the list?

Medical

Health Insurance: What is their health insurance plan? Are they on Medicare, available to all people sixty-five and over, and if so, do they have a supplemental plan? What all is included?

Medical Assistance (MA) or Medicaid: Only certain individuals can qualify for MA. Are they on MA, and if not, are they eligible? (People receiving MA must have a limited about of assets and have a medical necessity to qualify.) Can you find all of the "Important Documents" needed to apply for MA? You will need at least five years of documentation.

Medical Team: Do you have a list of your loved one's physicians or other medical professionals?

- Doctors
- Dentist
- Pharmacy
- Specialists
- Therapists
- Chiropractor

Veterans: Is your loved one a veteran? Do they access VA resources? If not, you may want to see what is available.

Legal

A qualified attorney can advise people on what is needed in their situation. They also know what is relevant for the state your loved one lives in. The following guidelines are informational only. It is important everyone have these documents in place (as applicable to their situation) and know and review these documents for your loved one.

Elder Care Attorney: A specific category of attorney specializing in the many legal impacts surrounding end of life.

Living Trust: This allows the transfer of assets without having to go through probate. Living trusts are expensive and may be complicated, but they are especially important for more complex situations, such as blended families, large estates, or remarriages.

Power of Attorney: This allows a designated individual to make decisions for a person on legal and financial matters. (Note a **durable power of attorney** remains in effect if the person becomes incapacitated.)

Will: Does your loved one have a will? Is it current and properly notarized or signed by two individuals as required by their state law? Who is the executor? Make certain they are still alive and willing to make decisions.

Healthcare Directive: Together, the power of attorney for healthcare and living will could be called a Healthcare Directive.

Living Will: This document allows the individual to indicate what type of care they might want should they become incapacitated or unable to decide for themselves. It often goes hand-in-hand with the power of attorney for healthcare.

The living will may contain a "Do-Not-Resuscitate" (DNR) order. Also, most hospitals and care homes require these documents to be available upon admission, or they will work with the patient to make one for that situation. The actual DNR decision will be made by a qualified physician.

Power of Attorney for Healthcare: Who will make decisions should the person be unable to make them for him or herself?

Even with these healthcare documents in place, you should have a verbal discussion with your loved one when they are capable of making decisions to hear firsthand what they desire at that point in life.

Overwhelmed? I encourage you to tackle a little bit at a time. Once you have all of the documents in a central location, you will be able to easily access them for future needs such as applying for benefits. The other benefit: you and your loved one will have more peace of mind about the future, and you just may avoid a financial or legal disaster.

Links to more caregiver resources can be found at nancyrpoland.com/caregiver-resources.

Appendix 2

Caregiving Checklist
for Home Care

If you are considering taking an aging or disabled family member into your home, review this checklist and honestly answer the questions.

1. What is your current relationship with your loved one? What is the relationship of other people in your household with the one who may move in? If there are current disagreements or tensions, will these be magnified when your loved one moves in?

2. Is everyone in your household "all in"? Will they support you? How will they contribute to the care of your loved one?

3. What has been done to assess the person's health status and by whom? What level of care do they need, and are you capable of providing the care?

4. What services will you need to outsource to help take care of your loved one?

5. What is your loved one's financial status? Will they be expected to contribute to the household expenses? Do they have resources to pay for extra care as needed?

6. Is this move expected to be temporary or permanent? Under what circumstances will the arrangement need to change?

7. Can you set good boundaries so that everyone in the household can still have a fulfilling existence?

8. What resources do you have in place for your own self-care?

9. What if your marriage suffers or your underage children are not getting enough care and attention? Will you be willing to end the caregiving for the sake of your family?

10. What modifications will need to be done to your home to accommodate your loved one? For example, will you need handles in the bathtub or a raised toilet seat? How will you get those things done?

11. Finally, are you physically, mentally, and emotionally up to the task?

These questions are just a start as there will be many more considerations on your caregiving journey. There are no right or wrong answers. Every family and every situation are different. As illustrated in Chapter 3: Life on Hold, it is important for a family to agree and have adequate resources when considering home care of a family member or other individual.

Appendix 3
Questions for Discussion

The following questions could be used by book clubs, caregiving groups, or other organizations discussing caregiving. The stories could be read individually over time or in a single session. There are individual questions for each chapter as well as general questions at the end.

Chapter 1: The Kidnapping Plot

1. Cynthia came from a large family. How were the caregiving duties shared between family members? Was this adequate? Could Cynthia have taken additional steps to involve her siblings, or would having more people involved create other problems?

2. Rob and Margaret moved to Missouri to enjoy their retirement. In spite of being a savvy businessman, Rob did not have the proper legal paperwork to allow his wife to be taken care of when he was not available. In hindsight,

how could Rob's children, and in particular Cynthia, have addressed this situation with her dad? Try role playing a "difficult conversation" regarding legal and financial issues.

3. How did Cynthia's can-do attitude help her caregiving? How did it make her life more difficult?

4. Do you think it was ethical for Cynthia to "kidnap" her mom and move her out of state? Why or why not? What could the outcome have been had she waited for all of the legalities to be in place?

Chapter 2: To Buddy with Love

1. How did Carol's upbringing affect the way she took care of Buddy? Did it help her not to be discouraged or pamper him too much?

2. At first, Landen tried to ignore Buddy because he did not want to deal with the possibility of losing his son. Do you see this as a sign of the times he lived in, the fact that he was the father, or his personality? How did his outlook turn around when Carol put her foot down, and how did Landen and Buddy's relationship evolve?

3. Considering the time period, could Carol have done more to get others involved in Buddy's care, especially when he was small?

4. Marcie and Buddy were close in age. When Marcie became an adult, she became an advocate for anyone with disabilities. Do you view this as something good coming out of a difficult situation? If so, how could other siblings of a child with challenges be taught to value the differences found in others?

Chapter 3: Life on Hold

1. Do you agree with Sandra and Ken's decision to care for Joe in their household right up to the end of his life? If no, what alternative would you have sought? If yes, do you think their care of him was adequate?

2. Evaluate Sandra's efforts to involve others in Joe's care-taking. Did she do a good job of seeking out resources? Is there anything she could have done differently?

3. Practice a conversation Sandra could have had with her dad when he was being too particular about his care or when he was being resistant about having others care for him. How might Joe have reacted, and what words could bring him around to Sandra's viewpoint?

4. Ken said he prayed about the decision to take in Joe. Do you believe God guides our decisions? What would Ken have done had he not felt they should take him in?

5. At the end, Joe had a fall where he had to be hospitalized, and he ultimately died. Does this change your ideas of taking care of a loved one at home?

Chapter 4: Friendship

1. What do you admire most about Phil's care for his friend? Did he do a good job balancing his friendship with Wally and the needs of Wally's wife, Kathleen?

2. How difficult do you think it was for Phil to ignore the manifestation of Wally's Parkinson's, for example watching him eat? What type of inner strength did it take for Phil to take Wally out in public when he was struggling?

3. When I asked Phil about the differences in caretaking for a man, he wanted to ensure he did not sound sexist. In general, do you agree with him that women are more into caregiving and men need to make more of an effort to be that type of caregiver? Generally speaking, what could be advantages to being a male in a caregiving situation?

4. Because more women than men get diseases such as Alzheimer's and women tend to live longer than men, there will likely be many more male caregivers in the future. Do you see this as a positive trend, a negative trend, or neutral? Why?

Chapter 5: Paradise Lost and Found

1. Jean's parents were from the southern part of the U.S. and moved to Gary, Indiana where they found success in the steel mills. How did her family or origin affect her future life? What values did she learn? How may her outlook have changed when the economy in Gary plunged?

2. Do you think Jean could have enlisted more help with taking care of her mom? Do you believe she placed care of her mom ahead of her own needs, and if so, why?

3. Jean was able to break out of the cycle of poverty by moving her family to Minneapolis. Do you see this as a brave move and something more people who find themselves in an economic downturn could do?

4. Whether inequality in healthcare is due to poverty—as in Jean's situation—race, or other factors, does this story help you have a better understanding of the devastation

of poor healthcare? What can you do to address this situation in our society?

Chapter 6: Finding Purpose in Pain

1. How would you have reacted receiving a dual diagnosis of Down syndrome and leukemia for your child within two days?
2. When Tyler was in the hospital being treated for leukemia, he nearly died. Miraculously, as his grandma held him, his fever came down and his blood pressure returned to normal. Do you believe this was a miracle from God? Do you think modern medical care leads to its own miracles? How do science and God interact?
3. What do you admire most about how this family turned tragedy into purpose?
4. What personal qualities does Angie have that led her to be a live-in host? If the circumstances were right, could you see yourself taking on that calling? Why or why not?

Overall Questions

1. What lesson(s) about caregiving did you take away from these stories?
2. If you had a friend or family member becoming exhausted and run down due to caretaking, how would you recommend they enlist help and resources?
3. Caregiving often involves difficult conversations about legal documents, finances, driving, and more. Talk about experiences where you had to have a difficult conversation and how you could have handled things differently.

If you did not practice one of these difficult conversations above, share a sentence or two you could use while taking to a loved one about needing to take care of legal or financial items.

4. How do you think faith plays a part in caregiving? Do you see a difference in people who believe in a higher power versus people who do not? How about people who believe in life after death versus people who think this world is the end?

5. Which of the six caregivers would you most like to meet? What qualities did he or she have that impressed you?

6. Pick one of the stories to discuss how caregiving made the caregiver a better person.

7. Pick one story to discuss if caregiving may have or could have resulted in a negative effect on the caregivers.

8. Did any of the stories make you uncomfortable? If yes, why?

9. If you were to find yourself in one of these caregiving situations, what are three steps you could take to ensure you maintain your mental, emotional, or physical health?

10. What other type of caregiving situations could be addressed in a book of this nature? Do you have a story to tell? If so, send your ideas to author@nancyrpoland.com.

Acknowledgments

Many people played a part in this story.

I am forever grateful to the six caregivers who freely shared their stories. Several others helped with the storytelling, adding depth and content.

My husband John has stood by me and cheered me on for over forty years. He is a caregiver by nature, and together we have weathered the ups and downs of life.

A heartful thank you to Nancy Muellner for the sketches. You added depth, beauty, and expression to the stories.

A special thank you to Terri Alston, who proofread this manuscript multiple times, and to readers Tery Blahut, Sue Flesch, and Marla Hartson, who provided content input. Thank you to those who took the time to read the book, and offered endorsements, and to Dr. Blight, who penned the foreword.

I am grateful to Meagan Thompson, my copy editor, who added polish and professionalism.

Gratitude to Brittany Miller of Brittany Cahoy Photography for the headshot.

Thank you to W. Terry Whalin and Morgan James Publishing for believing in me and providing guidance and support through every step.

Most of all, thanks be to God who has gifted us with the abilities needed to help others through the path of life.

Endnotes

1   AARP and National Alliance for Caregiving. Caregiving in
    the United States 2020. Washington, DC: AARP. May 2020.
2   Jean Accius, PhD, Spotlight 26, March 2017 Breaking
    Stereotypes: Spotlight on Male Family Caregivers, AARP
    Public Policy Institute
3   Wikipedia, Richard G. Hatcher and Wikipedia, Gary Works
4   2019 National Healthcare Quality and Disparities Report.
    Rockville, MD: Agency for Healthcare Research and Qual-
    ity; December 2020. AHRQ Pub. No. 20(21)-0045-EF

About the Author

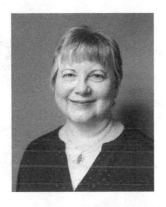

Nancy Poland approaches life with a mix of compassion and practicality. Through her experience as a caregiver for her premature son, a foster child, grandparents and parents, Nancy seeks to better the lives of caregivers and their loved ones through her writing and speaking. A life-long resident of Minneapolis and St. Paul, Minnesota, she and her husband John raised two sons and continue to contribute to their communities. Professionally Nancy manages proposals, contracts and grants; she has utilized her writing and negotiation skills to support both for-profit and non-profit companies. After finishing her master's degree in Health and Human Services Administration, Nancy wrote a thesis on privacy regulations and published an article in the National Contract Management magazine. She also writes stewardship materials, blogs, and communicates via social media through Nancy Poland and Grace's Message.

A free ebook edition is available with the purchase of this book.

To claim your free ebook edition:

1. Visit MorganJamesBOGO.com
2. Sign your name CLEARLY in the space
3. Complete the form and submit a photo of the entire copyright page
4. You or your friend can download the ebook to your preferred device

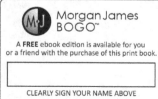

A **FREE** ebook edition is available for you or a friend with the purchase of this print book.

CLEARLY SIGN YOUR NAME ABOVE

Instructions to claim your free ebook edition:
1. Visit MorganJamesBOGO.com
2. Sign your name CLEARLY in the space above
3. Complete the form and submit a photo of this entire page
4. You or your friend can download the ebook to your preferred device

Print & Digital Together Forever.

Snap a photo

Free ebook

Read anywhere

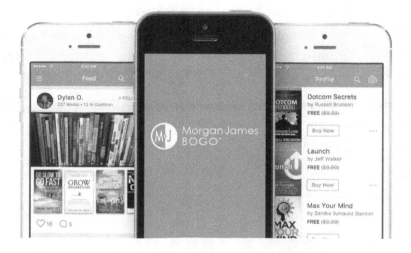

CPSIA information can be obtained
at www.ICGtesting.com
Printed in the USA
JSHW021257300123
37062JS00001B/56